CHAIR PILATES AND YOGA

Seated Exercises to Improve Strength, Flexibility, Balance and Posture

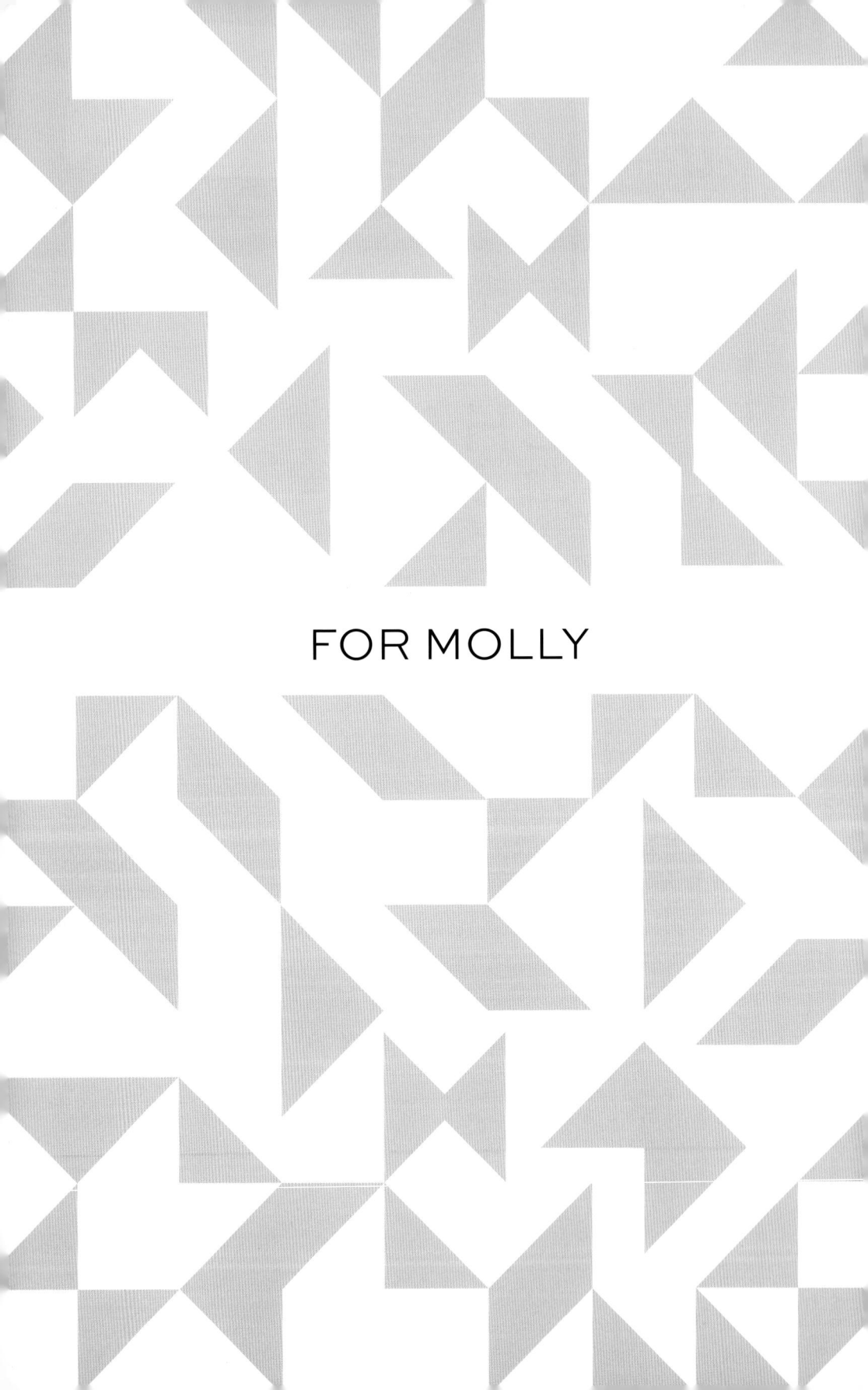

FOR MOLLY

CHAIR PILATES AND YOGA

Seated Exercises to Improve Strength, Flexibility, Balance and Posture

Harri Angell

GREEN TREE

LONDON • OXFORD • NEW YORK • NEW DELHI • SYDNEY

GREEN TREE
Bloomsbury Publishing Plc
50 Bedford Square, London, WC1B 3DP, UK
29 Earlsfort Terrace, Dublin 2, Ireland

BLOOMSBURY, GREEN TREE and the GREEN TREE logo are trademarks of
Bloomsbury Publishing Plc

First published in Great Britain 2024 by Bloomsbury Publishing Plc

A catalogue record for this book is available from the British Library

Library of Congress Cataloguing-in-Publication data has been applied for

ISBN (PB): 978-1-3994-1524-8

(epdf): 978-1-3994-1526-2

(epub): 978-1-3994-1525-5

2 4 6 8 10 9 7 5 3 1

Cover and inside studio photography by Henry Hunt
Images on following pages by Getty Images: 6, 8, 12, 15, 17, 19, 31, 34, 35, 42, 49, 69, 82, 86,
93, 96, 98, 113, 124, 127, 132, 146, 162, 171, 173, 179, 180

Geometric pattern design from Adobe Stock

Design by D.R. Ink

Printed and bound in China by RR Donnelley Asia Printing Solutions Limited

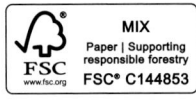

MIX
Paper | Supporting
responsible forestry
FSC® C144853

To find out more about our authors and books visit
www.bloomsbury.com and sign up for our newsletters

CONTENTS

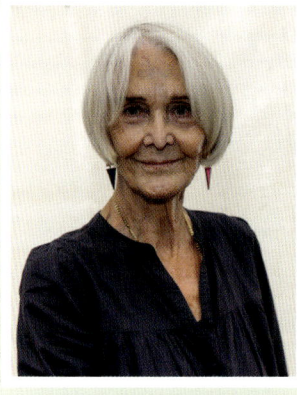

CASE STUDY

DAME SHEILA HANCOCK
AGE 92

'All my life, I have needed to keep fit and mobile. It is a prerequisite if you are doing eight performances a week dancing and singing in a musical, or enduring a 12-hour day filming. I had to climb a mountain for one film when I was 85.

I have done yoga, weights, a gym workout, running, and tap and ballet classes. In my ninth decade I have found these activities increasingly difficult. Then I came across Harri Angell's version of Chair Pilates and Yoga. Most of the exercises can be done sitting down, maybe whilst watching television if, like me, you find exercise boring. To begin with, they seemed laughably easy, but as I got more advanced, they demanded more, until I felt I was doing a strenuous workout — sitting down. The improvement in my strength, mobility and fluidity is remarkable. However rusty your body feels, I urge you to give it a try.'

INTRODUCTION

Welcome to *Chair Pilates and Yoga.*

Inside these pages, you will discover accessible, effective exercises that can be performed while seated and a few others that use the chair as a prop. The movements are, in the main, influenced by mat Pilates and yoga.

Chair Pilates and Yoga is an enjoyable, beneficial alternative to most traditional forms of exercise classes and routines that require you to get up and down from the floor. For some people, this just isn't possible. If you have mobility issues you might already find the thought of regular exercise challenging. Public classes can be intimidating, or perhaps you've given up on the idea of exercise altogether because you feel 'too old', 'too stiff', 'too unfit' and more!

I'm here to guide you through a number of simple, seated exercises that I promise will motivate you to keep going and get fitter. Ultimately all this will change how you feel. In addition, these exercises are portable: you can take them with you anywhere and perform them at any time; all you need is a chair. Sitting at home watching TV or listening to music, sitting in the garden or seated on a park bench, at the airport or a bus stop (ignore the stares!) — just take this book with you and you'll have some fitness routines at your fingertips.

I don't believe in age. I believe in energy. Don't let age dictate what you can or cannot do.'

Tao Porchon-Lynch (who taught yoga until her death at 101 years old)

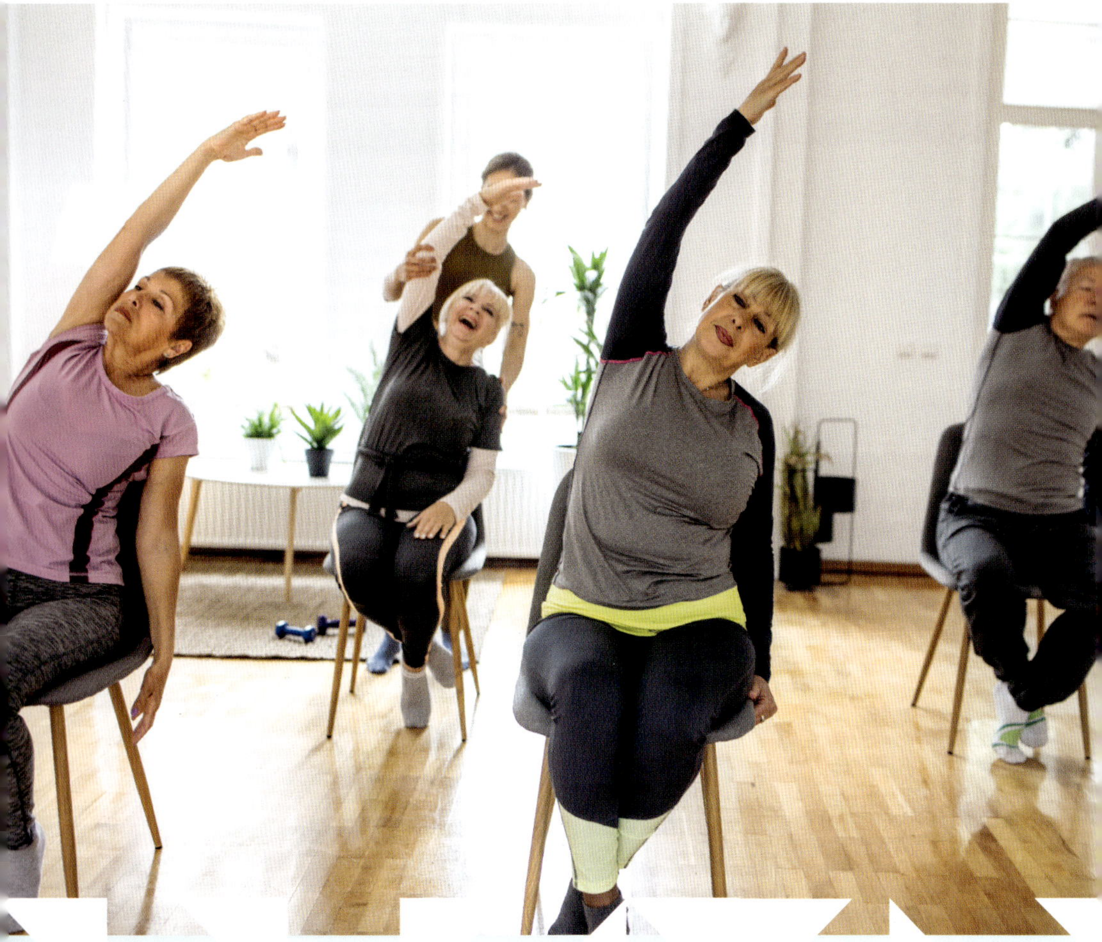

As we age, it's inevitable that changes take place in our bodies and minds. There's little we can do about our chronological age or our genetics, despite marketing promises that tell us we can 'turn back the clock' if we buy and use a super-duper product. However, what I believe we can do is slow down and actually influence the ageing process in a positive way. This will assist us to live well and have a healthy, happy later life.

The exercises will also benefit those of you who are recovering from an injury or illness and who need to take it slowly and gently while you mend. Sedentary office workers, too, will find a separate chapter (*see* p. 180) with simple exercise suggestions that can easily be fitted into a busy working day.

All that's required to achieve any of this is a commitment to put some time and effort into maintaining our bodies and minds as best we can. Everything you need to get moving is in this book. It's never, ever too late to start – let's challenge those ageist stereotypes now!

You'll find an abundance of exercises for all levels of fitness within these pages, set out in separate chapters for easy access to specific parts of the body. For example, if you wake up with a stiff neck, just turn to chapter 6, which contains all the neck exercises. However, before you start, it's probably a good idea to leaf through the book so that you become familiar with the chapters and the movements that suit your needs. Some I suggest you perform slowly with your breath, while others are slightly more dynamic and, in fact, I've included a faster 'cardio' routine towards the end of the book on page 156. It's up to you how many repetitions of the exercise you feel like completing. My suggestions are just that: suggestions. Listen to your body.

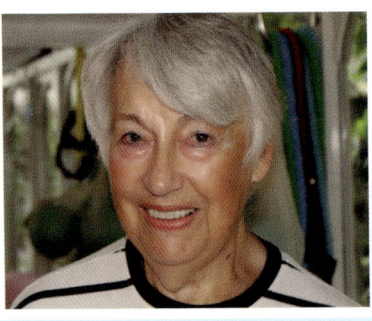

ANNIE BOVILL
AGE 89

'Throughout my life I've always done various keep-fit classes and then I took up Pilates, once a week, about 20 years ago. It particularly helped me after I got my new hips. This went on until Covid struck and then slowly arthritis and age began to catch up with me. First, my legs started to ache and then my balance got worse. Now I attend Harri's Chair Pilates and Yoga classes and they are helping me massively. I can stand better; my posture and balance are improving and I feel stronger and more confident. More than that, I am 90 next birthday and I can still manage to do all the seated exercises, and the old muscles still respond enough to keep me enjoying life and planning my 90th birthday party next year.'

NHS guidelines state that those of us over 65 should try to be physically active daily and aim to perform exercises that specifically improve flexibility, balance and strength on at least two days a week. Furthermore, the guidelines state that we do at least 150 minutes of activity a week at a moderate intensity or 75 minutes of activity at a higher intensity if we're already active. Finally, and this goes without saying, we should reduce time spent sitting or lying down for long periods.

If you haven't done any exercise for a while or feel nervous about your abilities, then stick to the ones marked beginner (B) or follow the beginner routine at the end of the book on page 185 to get you started. For those of you who feel ready for more challenging exercises then choose the ones marked intermediate (I).

I've been teaching Chair Pilates and Yoga to a number of people for some time, and you'll find their stories peppered throughout the book. You'll read how they have all benefited in different ways and discover that just because you're sitting down to exercise, it doesn't mean that you can't work hard — you can!

Good luck.

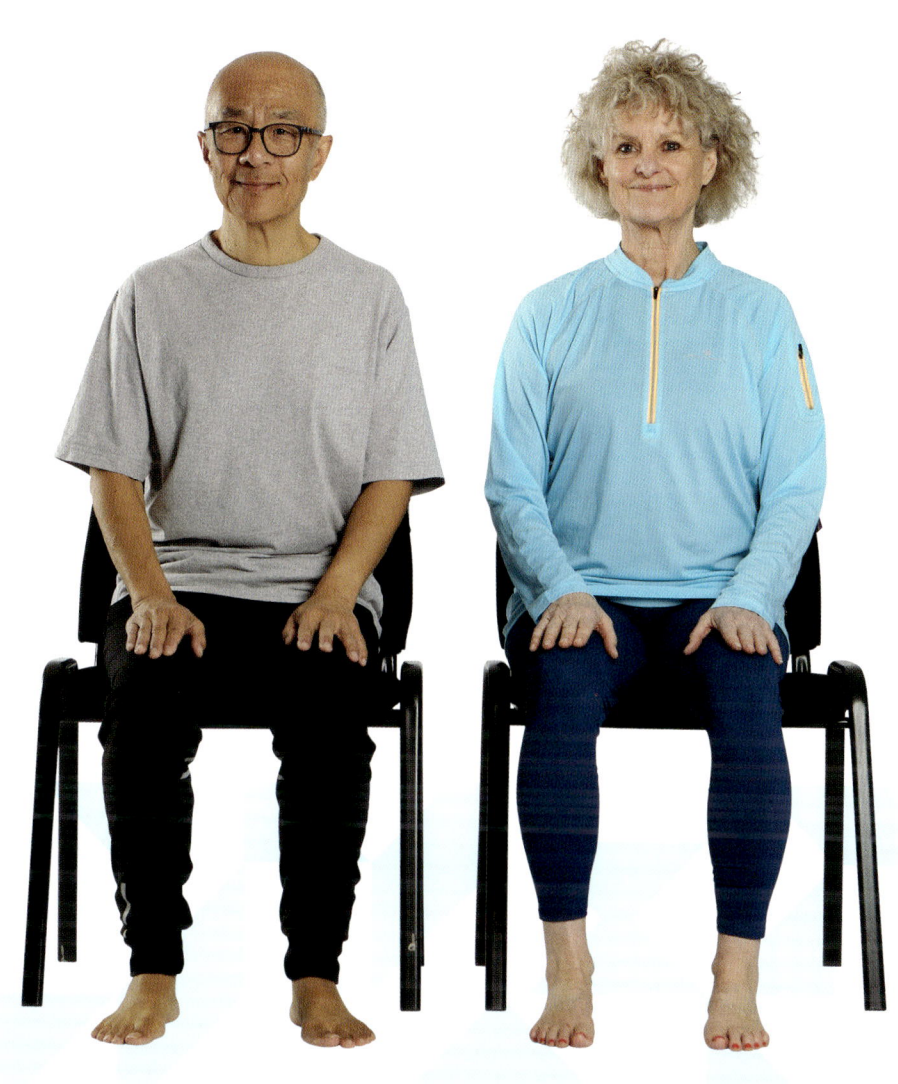

CHAPTER 1

WHAT CAN YOU EXPECT FROM CHAIR PILATES AND YOGA?

In the following chapters you'll find more detail about the countless benefits of a chair-based movement practice and why it is so important for us, at whatever age, to keep working on our strength, coordination, mobility, flexibility, balance, breathing, concentration and posture.

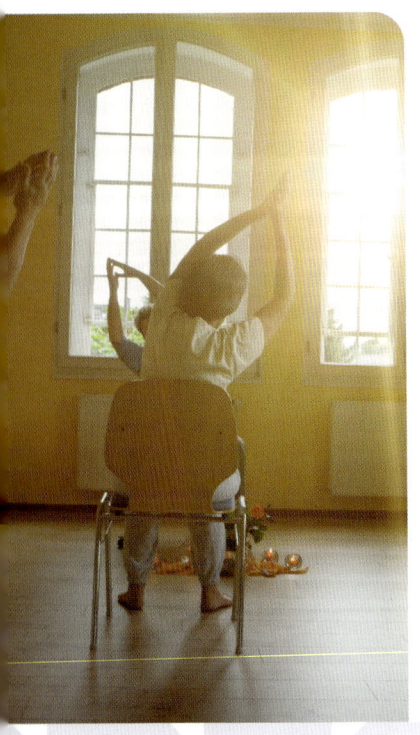

Your **strength** will improve – we lose approximately 3–8 per cent of our muscle mass per decade after the age of 30 and after the age of 60, the percentage is much higher.

This is not a very happy statistic. But all is not lost. The best way to fight this muscle loss is to keep using our muscles in order that they remain as strong and flexible as they possibly can. If you wish to, you can use small hand weights and/or ankle weights for some of the exercises; and there's a separate chapter about using a resistance band on page 141. Adding weight or resistance to your exercise session will make the movements slightly more challenging. But none of these extras are compulsory, so don't let that put you off; they're suggestions for when, or if, you feel ready or want a change. Always work in a way that is comfortable and safe for you.

You will also find improvement in your **coordination**, something that can begin to wander off and (literally) trip us up in our later years when our movements become slower and less smooth. Practice will keep it alive.

Your **mobility** will become smoother. It's hard, I know, to get going when your joints or muscles ache and you have no energy or motivation to do so. But move, we must. Seated exercise makes it all much easier and achievable, and I think you'll be pleasantly surprised by how your mobility can change for the better. This improvement can have a positive effect not only on your body but also on your mind – all while sitting down.

Additionally, there will be noticeable gains in your **flexibility**. With some simple, gentle stretch exercises, those annoying tight muscles will thank you – I so often hear, 'I'm not flexible, I can't do yoga or Pilates.' It doesn't matter; you just stretch your body to wherever your own physical point of tension is reached. It's all relative, and over time, you will feel, and even see, your flexibility increase, which in turn will help you move more easily. There's a separate chapter (see p. 162) just for stretching, but you'll find many of the general exercises in this book incorporate stretching that will improve your flexibility, too.

A very important aspect of our later lives is being able to **balance**, and because of this, you'll find a whole chapter dedicated to balance on page 132. Preventing falls as we grow older is vital, but sadly our ability to balance decreases as we age, so once again, practice is important. One of the things I suggest you do regularly is stand on one leg while holding on to the back of the chair for safety, and I will explain more about this, and all the other improvements that relate to balance, later on.

Breathing – this is not something we're necessarily conscious of, and mostly we take it for granted, but our lungs are muscles too and need to be used to their full capacity to keep working well. Breathing deeply can be relaxing, and I will explain how a breathing and relaxation practice can be of real benefit on page 28. I've also included a short, mindful breathing exercise on page 178.

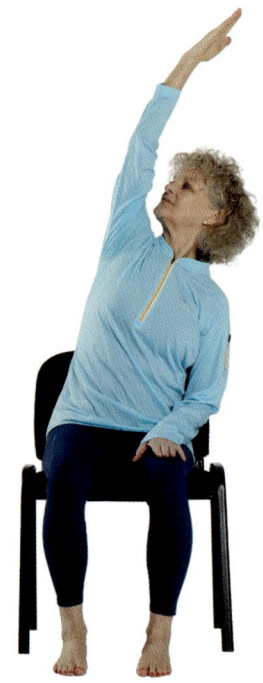

The more efficiently you breathe, the more your body is oxygenated and the better you will feel.

Good **concentration** is something else that becomes more of a challenge as we age. Learning to focus on the movements as you perform them along with the breathing can increase your ability to concentrate. As a result, you'll also find that you're more alert. Cognitive problems, including loss of good concentration can be caused by sleep deprivation. There's a chapter on sleep with suggestions about how you can relax, with a couple of wonderful yoga routines (Restorative Yoga and Yoga Nidra, *see* pp. 173 and 176) to have a better quality of sleep.

Your **posture** will improve. You'll notice that you begin to sit and stand up straighter and move through your day more easily. Walking without assistance and maintaining a healthy walking gait for as long as possible is the aim. Frailty can creep up on us, but don't let it surprise you; keep your body and mind active and it won't catch you out.

The proportion of people who are physically inactive increases sharply with age, particularly after the age of 55. The increase in physical activity we had seen in recent years among those aged 75 and over has been lost during the pandemic.'

The State of Ageing 2022 report, Centre for Ageing Better

And finally, what this book and all these exercises that are influenced by Pilates and yoga can provide you with, is an overall sense of **well-being and zest for life**. Whatever your age, state of health or outlook, renewed energy, increased independence, purpose and joy can become yours with just a little time spent every day on some of these simple exercises.

For a more detailed explanation of the benefits gained from Chair Pilates and Yoga, see chapter 3 on page 20.

Traditionally Pilates and yoga are taught standing up or lying down. The exercises in this book are adaptations rather than the true movements of both disciplines, and the exercises, as I said earlier, are influenced by both these rewarding practices.

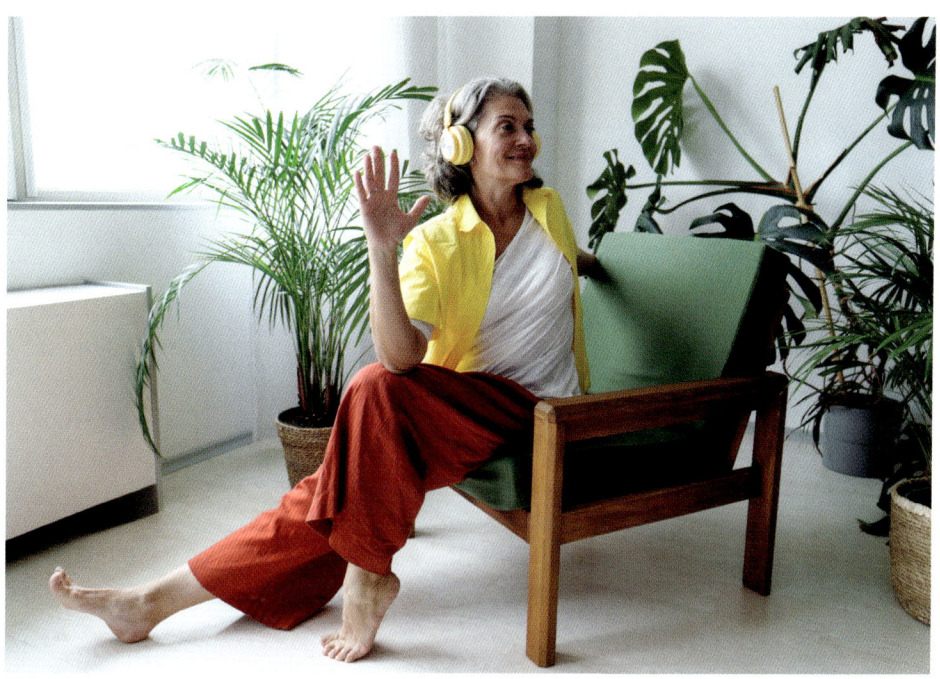

However, the principles of Pilates and yoga still stand.

You'll find some of the exercises and chapters start with a brief explanation of how the movements benefit us as we age. I think it helps to know why you're doing an exercise and how it can improve your fitness levels, particularly if you want to target one area of your body that is weak or needs, for whatever reason, to be woken up or stretched. One thing that happens when we grow older is that we can lose touch with our bodies. Perhaps this is because we begin to feel less attractive, frailer and not as able as we used to be. This can then lead to a loss of confidence. Sadly, society as a whole doesn't do much to help the older community feel particularly useful or visible. But I believe, with a little guidance, we can create this for ourselves.

I hope that these exercises will encourage you to reconnect with your body; after all, it's been doing a pretty good job for many years. I hope too that you can regain a sense of self and confidence if you currently find this lacking.

You'll find expert advice from a couple of general practitioners, an osteopath, and a physiotherapist who works specifically with older people, peppered throughout. **However, and this is important: if you're not sure about the suitability of these exercises for you please take medical advice from a health professional before attempting any of them, particularly if you are post-operative.**

Although this book is aimed at an older audience, younger people can, of course, benefit, too. Included is a chapter on a desk workout for those who find themselves in a sedentary job, sitting in front of a computer (on a chair!) all day with little movement in their life (*see* p. 180). The exercise routines might also be useful for those of you who are maybe struggling with particular health issues — long Covid, type 2 diabetes, cancer, rheumatoid arthritis or Parkinson's, for example.

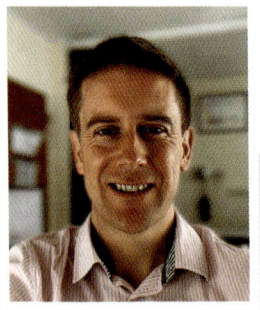

PROFESSIONAL ADVICE

DR MATTHEW ROBINSON
GENERAL PRACTITIONER

Matthew says:

'Regular physical activity is part of the routine care of type 2 diabetes. Regular exercise and, in particular, increasing muscle bulk improves the way our bodies respond to the hormone insulin (problems with which are the main cause of this condition). Increasing muscle mass helps move sugar out of the bloodstream so it can be safely stored.

Physical activity helps to reduce our blood pressure and cholesterol levels (both important in diabetes and preventing heart attacks and strokes) as well as helping us to lose weight, probably the most important thing we can do in controlling type 2 diabetes. Increasingly we are seeing people manage their type 2 diabetes so well that they put it into remission and physical activity can be an important part of this.'

CHAPTER 2

A BRIEF HISTORY OF PILATES AND YOGA

PILATES

Joseph Pilates was born in 1883 in Germany. As a child, he suffered from rickets, asthma and rheumatic fever. Frustrated by his frailty he explored ways to improve his health and physical fitness and eventually became a gymnast, skier, boxer, diver and bodybuilder while also studying self-defence and meditation.

In 1912 Joseph Pilates moved to England to teach self-defence to members of the British police force and army. When World War I broke out he was interned in Knockaloe Camp on the Isle of Man, where he refined his exercise techniques using all he had learned from yoga, gymnastics, self-defence, weight training and martial arts.

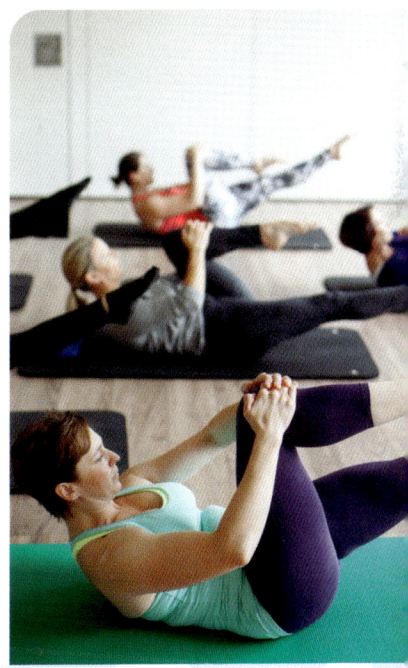

Calling this method of body conditioning 'Contrology', Pilates observed that if a body was misaligned or weak in a particular area, the muscles and joints would overcompensate, often causing injuries, so he continued to develop his exercises, concentrating on physical remedies for postural misalignments.

> It is indeed true that by practising yoga we gradually improve our ability to concentrate and to be independent. We improve our health, our relationships, and everything we do.'
>
> T.K.V. Desikachar

On the ship emigrating to America after the war he met his future wife, Clara, who coincidentally shared his passion for fitness. In New York, together they set up a fitness studio. They trained actors, dancers and athletes to develop core strength, and the Pilates method became well known for rehabilitating those with injuries.

He passed on the Pilates method by teaching apprentices his programme of exercise, which continues to develop globally. Many of these 'Pilates Elders' went on to live long, healthy lives – a testament to the power of Pilates.

YOGA

Unlike Pilates, yoga has been around for thousands of years and its history is far more involved and, dare I say it, fascinating, than the history of Pilates. Joseph Pilates borrowed many yoga asanas (postures) and adapted them to suit his Pilates repertoire. However, yoga is so much more than just postures.

Yoga is an ancient Indian discipline that harnesses body, mind and spirit, and the word *yoga* actually means 'union' in Sanskrit – the mind and body coming together as one. There are many different variations and schools of yoga to choose from, and these are practised all over the world. The study of this ancient discipline can be a rewarding and sometimes life-changing experience.

Like Pilates, yoga can increase strength, coordination and flexibility and improve balance. It is also a very calming practice that can help you to fully relax both mentally and physically. The ancient philosophy of yoga and the breath practices (pranayama) can provide a powerful insight into who we are and why we are here.

Both these disciplines have influenced the chair exercises, and the benefits of combining the two, while seated, will pay dividends. Later on in the book, as I've already mentioned, there is a section on relaxation and breathing as an aid to sleeping well. This will invite you to try yoga nidra, often referred to as 'sleep yoga' because it can help you reach the wonderful state of consciousness between waking and sleeping. Also using the chair as a prop, I've included a couple of restful restorative yoga poses that can relieve stress, calm your body, rest tired legs and hopefully encourage good sleep. There is more about both of these on pages 173–8.

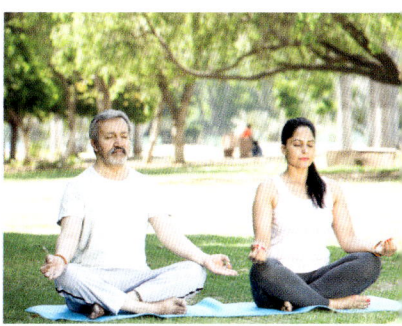

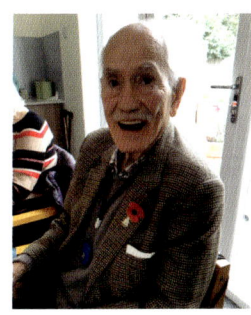

CASE STUDY

JOHN STEVENS
AGE 90

'I used to be a boxer; stopped when I was 60. I miss it and watch it on the TV and often think "I could have put him away!" I've always done sports. I held the record for the deepest dive, taught diving. Now, I keep independent, always moving; chucked the nurses out who came to help me! Once I stop moving, I get wobbly and stiff; exercise is good for me. I have to make sure I do it; that's why seated exercise is so good. I don't move one of my shoulders now: snapped a tendon and the other one is damaged from a fall. My legs don't straighten either, so I have to stand slowly; other than that I'm pretty fit! If I get an achy back, I do the seated roll down every three to four hours, which helps enormously, and when I watch TV, I rest my feet on a foot stool and do the feet exercises and ankle rotations. I was in a prisoner of war camp when I was younger and I thought I'd die young, but here I am at 90 and still going strong!'

CHAPTER 3

HOW CHAIR PILATES AND YOGA CAN HELP YOU

In chapter 1, I briefly touched on the benefits of the activities in this book and what they can do for you. In this chapter I will go into more detail – I'll take a look at the thinking behind Pilates and yoga and briefly examine the anatomy and physiology of our body in relation to the exercises.

POSTURE

Good posture – how you hold your body against gravity when moving about or walking – is vital for you to continue to use your body efficiently and with ease into your later life. When your posture is good, there is less strain on the joints and bones because they are held in correct alignment and you're not slouched, leaning or hunched.

Good posture can be successfully acquired only when the entire mechanism of the body is under perfect control. Graceful carriage follows as a matter of course.'

Joseph Pilates

Ageing can sometimes leave us feeling invisible to the world and, unfortunately, if we're not careful, our posture can reflect this feeling as we disappear into ourselves. By maintaining a good posture, we can stand tall and our muscles will remain lengthened and strong. Our legs and arms will be free to work at comfortably propelling us forwards as we move about or walk. How often do we see older people depicted as frail, hunchbacked shufflers? We need to try to end that image now and consciously work towards lengthening through the spine and walking tall, pain-free and proud.

How do you walk? Do you lift your head up and look forwards, towards the horizon? Do you shuffle? Or lift up your feet? What are your arms doing? Are your fists clenched? Are you lopsided? If you sit all day, then maybe you have a tendency to be round-shouldered and have tight hip flexors as well — hip flexors are at the top of your legs and help lift your leg up as you walk. Or maybe your knees ache, or you're unhappy in pain, or wear uncomfortable shoes, or walk with a limp — everything can affect your posture, which can then influence the way you feel. In addition, anxieties can turn into tension, and unresolved emotions can manifest themselves in stress-related niggles or injuries. So it's not surprising that we end up with a body that compensates and then starts to complain as the years progress into our later life.

Posture can also affect our well-being; standing upright — lengthening through the spine with an open chest and relaxed shoulders — immediately feels better than being slouched and scrunched up in a defeated, collapsed stance.

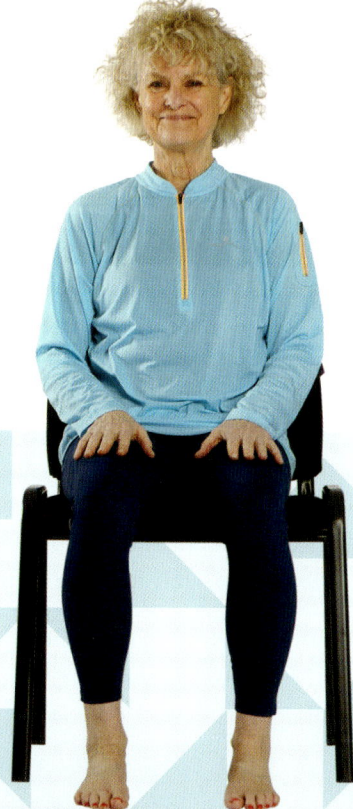

As we age our posture can obviously change, so it's important to start looking after it and become body-aware as early as possible. With good posture, all your vital organs will be held in the right place, everything will function well and you will move so much more easily and freely as you go about your everyday life and activities.

You'll find that before every exercise in this book, I say, 'Sit up tall, lengthen through the spine with your feet on the floor directly below your knees, and engage your abdominal muscles and/or pelvic floor muscles.' (More about this on page 24.) Getting into the habit of doing this will make such a difference to your posture and how you feel.

THE SPINE

When we move, our body is supported by the spine. It keeps us upright and carries the weight of our head, torso and arms. Good, upright walking and learning to keep the spine in its strongest, safest position, with the least stress placed on discs and ligaments, will make all the difference to your body and how you feel. Alignment is everything. The lower spine, the lumber region, is often where most people find they get discomfort as they age, whereas the middle and upper back, the thoracic spine, is where we can most often develop a round-shouldered hunch. We want to avoid both of these.

NEUTRAL SPINE

All exercises, it is advised, should start from a neutral spine position, usually when standing or lying down on the mat, but we are going to practise it seated on a chair. A neutral spine is important because it is a good, strong, healthy position for your spine to be in during movement and something that is worth noting and aiming for to avoid lower back aches and round shoulders. A neutral spine keeps the spine and pelvis aligned and arranged in their strongest position and in their natural curves, with the least amount of stress placed on discs and ligaments, which means you are less likely to injure yourself or get an aching back.

Your pelvis can tilt backwards and forwards but what we want is for your pelvis and spine to be as aligned as possible, not forwards or backwards, and this should feel natural.

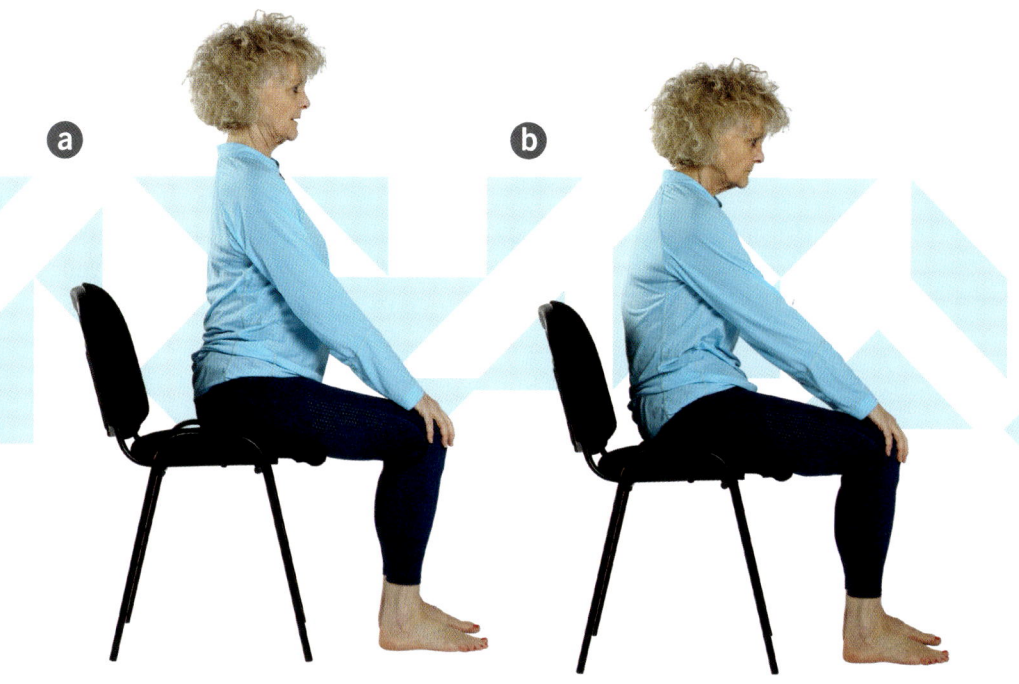

FINDING YOUR NEUTRAL SPINE WHILE SEATED

Method

Sit up tall on your chair, lengthen through the spine with your feet parallel on the floor below your knees. Place your hands on your hips and gently tilt your pelvis backwards and forwards — feel the small movement under your hands.

This visualisation can help: imagine your pelvis is a bowl of water. When you tilt your pelvis forwards (an anterior pelvic tilt, see image a), the water from the bowl spills out the front. When you tilt your pelvis backwards (a posterior pelvic tilt, see image b), the water from the bowl spills out the back. You'll also find that as you tilt your pelvis backwards your torso tends to collapse in its centre making it harder to sit up straight and tall. Bring the pelvis/bowl to a central position where the imaginary water stays level and doesn't spill. That's a neutral spine position and it should feel comfortable, not forced.

CORE MUSCLES AND ENGAGING YOUR ABDOMINAL AND PELVIC FLOOR MUSCLES

If you've ever attended a Pilates class, you will probably have heard the expression 'core' or 'powerhouse'. In yoga, too, the core muscles are often mentioned in relation to the muscles of the torso. Basically, your core is indeed your torso, the central part of your body, including your hips, abdomen, lower back and pelvis.

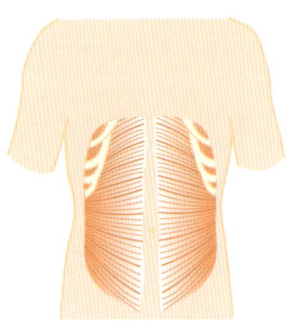

The transversus abdominis – this deep corset-like muscle wraps around our middle and works with the pelvic floor muscles to support the pelvis and spine – it's the one we need to engage when performing the exercises.

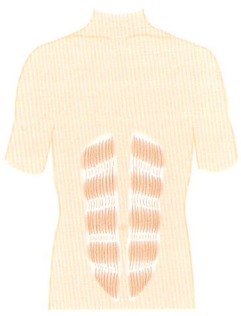

The rectus abdominis – our potential 'six pack'! It's never too late…

ENGAGING YOUR ABDOMINAL MUSCLES

Your abdominal muscles, specifically the deepest, corset-like one, which is called the transversus abdominis (TVA), wraps around your middle between your lower ribs and the top of your pelvis. These muscles work together with your pelvic floor muscles (*see* p. 26). Both sets of muscles support the pelvis and spine by maintaining something called intra-abdominal pressure during any exertion. If you suffer from back problems – which can sometimes creep up on us in later life, especially lower back ache, as mentioned in the explanation of the spine on page 22, which can also be caused by sitting a lot – it can often be because this corset-like abdominal muscle, the TVA, is weak.

When practising the exercises in this book, and in order to get the most out of the movements, it's a good idea to pull or engage your deep abdominal muscle (TVA) along with your pelvic floor muscles before you move.

When you first start trying out the exercises in this book, you may find it really hard to do both at the same time along with remembering which arm or leg you're meant to be lifting, and whether you're meant to be breathing in or out! Although in the written instructions for the exercises I remind you to engage your tummy muscles and pelvic floor muscles, you can just choose one when you're starting out — take your time to experiment and get to know how each contraction (the pulling in of your abdominal muscles and the pulling up of your pelvic floor) feels and what difference this can make to the execution of the movement.

The following visualisation and exercise are how I teach my clients to get in touch with their deep abdominal muscles and engage them, so have a go.

- Imagine you have a big belt wrapped around your waist. The belt has 10 notches.
- Visualise pulling the belt to the 10th notch so that your abdomen is pulled right in as far as it will go — not very comfortable or realistic and that is way too far!
- Relax the muscles.
- Now pull the imaginary belt halfway to the 5th notch. This is a bit more comfortable for your abdominal muscles.
- Relax the muscles.
- Now pull the imaginary belt to the 3rd notch.
- Generally, this is where you want to be pulling your abdominal muscles into each time you perform the exercise, the 3rd notch on your imaginary belt.

When you are doing this, you are supporting and stabilising your spine, immediately making your torso stronger, which in turn makes it easier to move your arms and legs because they have a secure and solid base from which to work.

GLUTES

These are your buttock muscles; they are also important core muscles, which need to stay strong for you to walk efficiently and climb stairs. Your glutes can also impact the hips and the lower back. If you sit all day then these, like other muscles, will weaken (and yes, we are going to be sitting when we perform most of the exercises in this book, but you can still work those bottom muscles!).

PELVIC FLOOR MUSCLES

As we age and lose muscle mass, our collagen begins to deplete — and for women, pregnancy and childbirth are an additional factor — and our pelvic floor muscles weaken.

Alongside the TVA, the pelvic floor muscles work to help stabilise and support the spine and pelvis by maintaining intra-abdominal pressure during exertion. Walking can increase intra-abdominal pressure, so a weak pelvic floor can lead to all sorts of problems for both men and women. The exercises in this book are an excellent way to strengthen the pelvic floor muscles to prevent urinary incontinence — so if yours is weak and you have problems as a result, these exercises can begin to fix it. But you will need to engage the muscle; it won't happen by magic. Below is a description of the way I instruct the clients in my classes.

To contract your pelvic floor muscles, the simplest way I find to describe it is to imagine stopping the flow of urine when you go for a wee. This applies to both men and women. Or imagine trying to stop breaking wind in public, by lifting up your back passage.

You may notice as you pull your pelvic floor muscles up that your deep TVA muscle activates at the same time — try it again now as you're reading this — proof if you need it that these two sets of muscles work together to support the spine and stabilise the pelvis. But more importantly, we can strengthen our pelvic floor muscles and avoid incontinence in our later life.

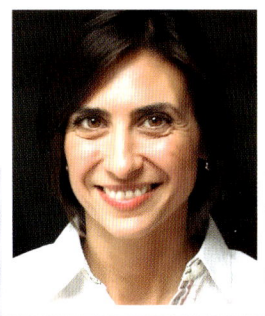

PROFESSIONAL ADVICE

DR HELEN KENNEDY
GENERAL PRACTITIONER

Helen, who has a special interest in women's health, describes the pelvic floor and talks about the benefits of pelvic floor exercises as we age:

'The pelvic floor is a sheet of muscle and connective tissue that spans the area underneath the pelvis, providing support to the pelvic organs including the bladder, bowel and, in women, the womb. If there is not adequate support, it can lead to prolapse and also lead to stress incontinence, which is where leakage of urine occurs with coughing, sneezing, jumping, or any activity that leads to a rise in pressure in the abdomen.

As we age, it is common for the pelvic floor to weaken, often for a combination of reasons. Having children can cause problems later in life and make us more prone to prolapse and urinary incontinence. Even without a difficult vaginal delivery, just the weight of carrying round a baby during pregnancy can weaken the pelvic floor. Another important factor can be the menopause when we experience declining levels of oestrogen, which is important in maintaining the quality and strength of muscle and connective tissue.

There is good evidence that pelvic floor exercises are beneficial in the management of urinary incontinence in women and [they] are used as a first line of treatment before other options such as surgery are considered. Up to 70 per cent improvement can be seen in symptoms when exercises are done correctly and consistently. The exercises can also be helpful in improving symptoms of prolapse. Specialist physiotherapy may be offered to those with more severe problems, but having an awareness of your pelvic floor through practising Chair Pilates and Yoga will undoubtedly be beneficial. Strengthening and pulling up that muscle "sling" will lift the pelvic organs and keep them where they are meant to be and work best.'

BREATHING

Before any real benefit can be derived from physical exercises, one must first learn how to breathe properly. Our very life depends on it.'

Joseph Pilates

Breathing while performing the exercises is another important aspect of the routines in this book for many different reasons, some of which I've already explained in the introduction (see p. 13). There is a tendency to hold your breath when concentrating, especially when you've not only got to think about the movements you need to make, but also think about pulling your abdominal muscles in and/or engaging your pelvic floor muscles. But learning to breathe, to focus on the breath as we move, can have an enormous impact on the way we feel and how we execute the exercise.

Breathing well during your chair practice will help to strengthen your diaphragm, which, in fact, does 80 per cent of the breathing work — we can't make our lungs any bigger, but we can improve our posture to help those lungs and diaphragm function more efficiently, which will also improve our overall stamina and how we feel as we grow older.

When we become physically or mentally tired, we tend to collapse from our centre, bend slightly in our middle and turn our torso into a C shape, which means we run the risk of becoming, over time, round-shouldered. This curved, C-like posture restricts the movement of the diaphragm and lungs. Good lung capacity enables us to transfer maximum oxygen into our body and muscles in order to optimise whatever activity we are doing. We need to be able to use our lungs fully and expand our rib cage comfortably, utilising the diaphragm to power our breathing.

You'll find that I include a lot of breathing cues for some of the exercises, encouraging you to use your breath in a specific way, but in other exercises, I just remind you to breathe in whatever way suits you.

Some exercises will require you to breathe in before you move, while others will ask you to breathe in as you make the movement. Take your time to master the breathing techniques and eventually everything will slot into place and become second nature. But the most important thing of all is not to hold your breath!

The breathing we use in Pilates is known as lateral thoracic breathing. If you decide to explore yoga further, you'll discover there are many breathing techniques (pranayama), the different practices of which can be immensely rewarding. There is more about breathing in relation to relaxation towards the end of this book, with a short mindful breathing exercise for you to try on page 178. By focusing on our breath we can help settle the mind and remove it from its daily chitter-chatter, which allows for stillness and peace – more on this later. For the purpose of this chair practice, we're going to keep it simple and concentrate on one form of breathing – lateral thoracic breathing. This type of breathing encourages you to breathe into your ribcage rather than into your belly, so that, ideally, you are able to activate your abdominal muscles at the same time.

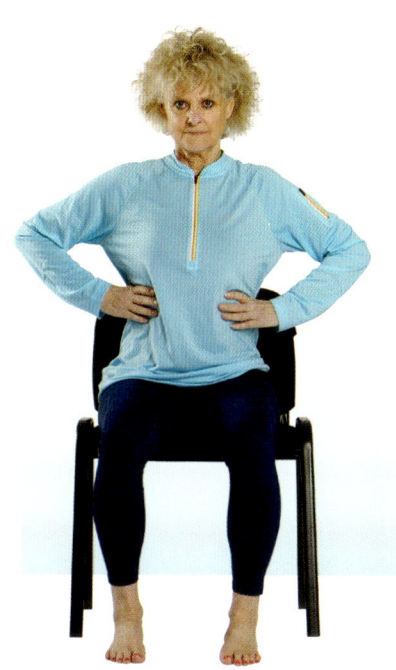

Method

- Sit up tall, lengthen through the spine with your feet on the floor below your knees.
- Place your hands on either side of your torso on your rib cage.
- Take a breath in through your nose and feel how the rib cage expands underneath your hands as you do so.
- Breathe out slowly through your mouth, allowing your rib cage to relax.
- Try not to let your shoulders rise up when you breathe in, as they tend to want to join in.

Aside from the health benefits of breathing well and using the lungs to their full capacity, this lateral thoracic breathing helps the exercises flow. If this is too challenging to begin with, just remember to breathe – that's all you need to do!

BALANCE

In order to balance well we need to develop something called proprioception: the ability to sense the position, location and orientation of your limbs in space. This skill doesn't happen by magic and, unfortunately, as we age, we begin to lose our ability to balance, which makes us more susceptible to falls and injuries that could otherwise be prevented. So it is absolutely essential that we keep practising it, every day if possible, and safely. You'll find balance exercises in chapter 17 from page 132.

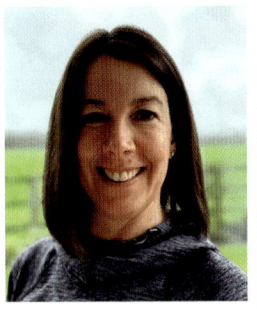

PROFESSIONAL ADVICE

SARA CARTER
PHYSIOTHERAPIST

Sara who works with older adults says:
'Anyone can have a fall, but as we get older our risk of falling increases. This can be for a number of reasons and often it's a combination of factors. One of the areas that we can control to reduce our risk is to ensure that we keep our muscles strong and joints as mobile as possible. Incorporating exercise into our daily routine is a key element of this; finding what works for you and your lifestyle is important to ensure the activity is ongoing. Chair Pilates and Yoga is something that most people find accessible and manageable within their normal routine.'

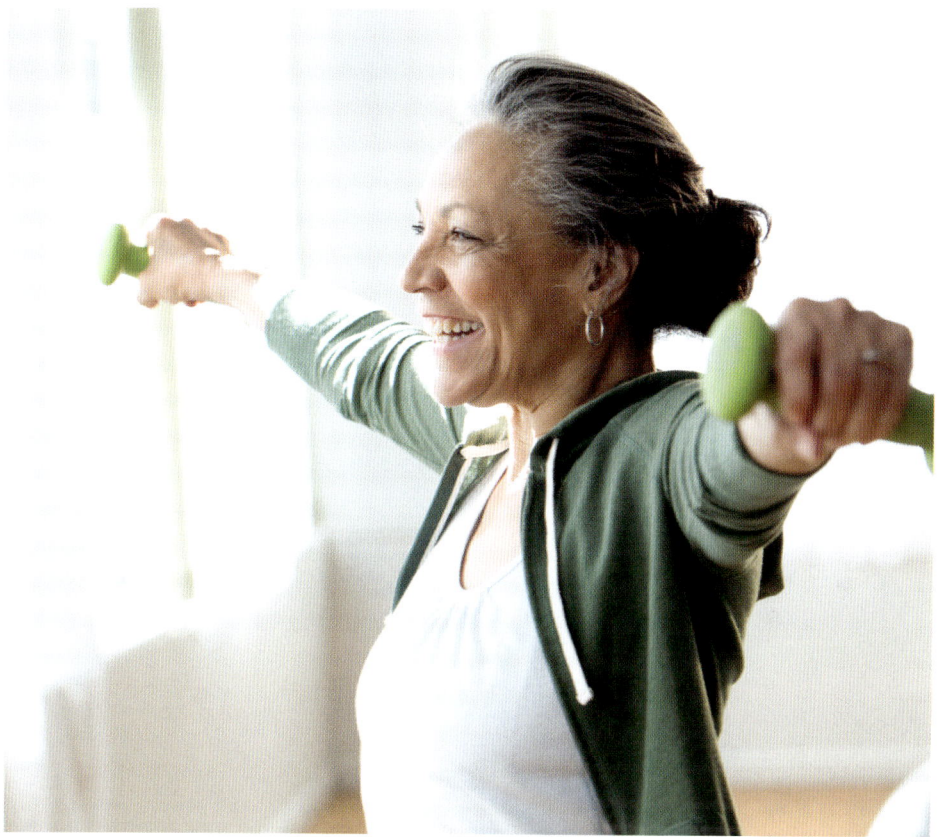

What also happens when our balance deteriorates, is we develop fear — fear of slips, tripping and walking on uneven surfaces, for example. This can sometimes force us to withdraw from social activities and prevent us from leaving the house. As we age socialising is important for our sense of overall well-being and is something to be nurtured, so practise your balancing, which will enable you to stay upright and to keep enjoying doing the things that you've always enjoyed doing.

COORDINATION

When we move about or walk, we need to coordinate our arm and leg movements and be conscious of our intentions, sometimes referred to as kinaesthetic sensing (the ability to feel movements of the limbs and body). Remember the 'rub your tummy, pat your head' game? That's coordination. This is another skill that tends to diminish in later life, which again, like balance, has implications for injuries and falls that end up making us frightened to venture out. Many of the exercises in this book will improve your coordination.

FLEXIBILITY

As we grow older and as a natural part of the ageing process, our joints tend to get stiffer and our muscles begin to lose their elasticity. But we can do something about this — become more active! If your muscles remain shortened, not stretched, which they will do if you sit all day and don't move around much, they can become tight and begin to weaken. Niggles can develop and injury can follow. In order that we retain full, comfortable mobility as we age in our day-to-day living, we need our muscles to be long. Remaining flexible will help with your balance, too — everything leads to balancing well!

CONCENTRATION

The ability to concentrate and focus can change as we get older — it's all part of a natural (and annoying) cognitive decline that happens over time. We tend to get more distracted too. But the good news is that by performing the exercises in this book and learning to concentrate on the moves, we can improve this skill — in the same way that our muscle strength improves with exercise, our brain function can improve with stimulation. Being able to apply oneself wholly to the task in hand and block out distractions isn't easy at the best of times. Once you are familiar with the exercises in this book, or those exercises that work for you, you'll find it easier to focus fully on each movement to get the most out of them. They'll become second nature to you. Try not to let your mind wander, ignore your 'to-do' list, switch off your phone and any other distractions and instead begin to feel the connection between concentrating your mind and the movements of your body. This will then transfer into your everyday life.

STAMINA

I often hear the cry, 'I'm too tired to exercise, I have no energy any more.' This can become a vicious circle: by not exercising because you feel too tired, your muscles will weaken and lethargy can set in making you even more tired than you already were! By working your muscles when practising the exercises in this book, slowly increasing the repetitions and trying out more challenging movements, you will be building strength and, in turn, increasing your stamina. Including seated exercise in your daily or weekly routine will pay dividends to how you feel. And of course, this transfers to your everyday activities: the stronger you become the more you'll build resistance to any niggles that might be lurking and be able to comfortably and safely sustain or return to whatever it is you choose to do as you age.

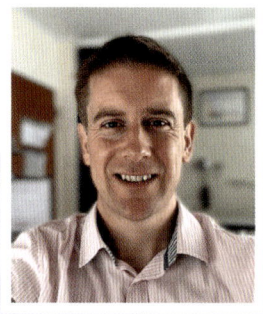

PROFESSIONAL ADVICE

DR MATTHEW ROBINSON
GENERAL PRACTITIONER

Matthew says:

'We have known for a long time that keeping active and mobile has significant benefits for our health. These benefits become more important as we get older, and we are faced with more challenges to our health, mobility and independence.

Regular exercise reduces the risk of heart disease and strokes, type 2 diabetes, breast and bowel cancer, depression and dementia. It protects against the risk of falls and improves the strength of our bones and reduces frailty.

It is recommended that those over 65 are active daily to improve balance, muscle strength and coordination. Even small increases in activity are known to be beneficial. As the saying goes, "We don't stop doing things because we get old; we get old because we stop doing things."'

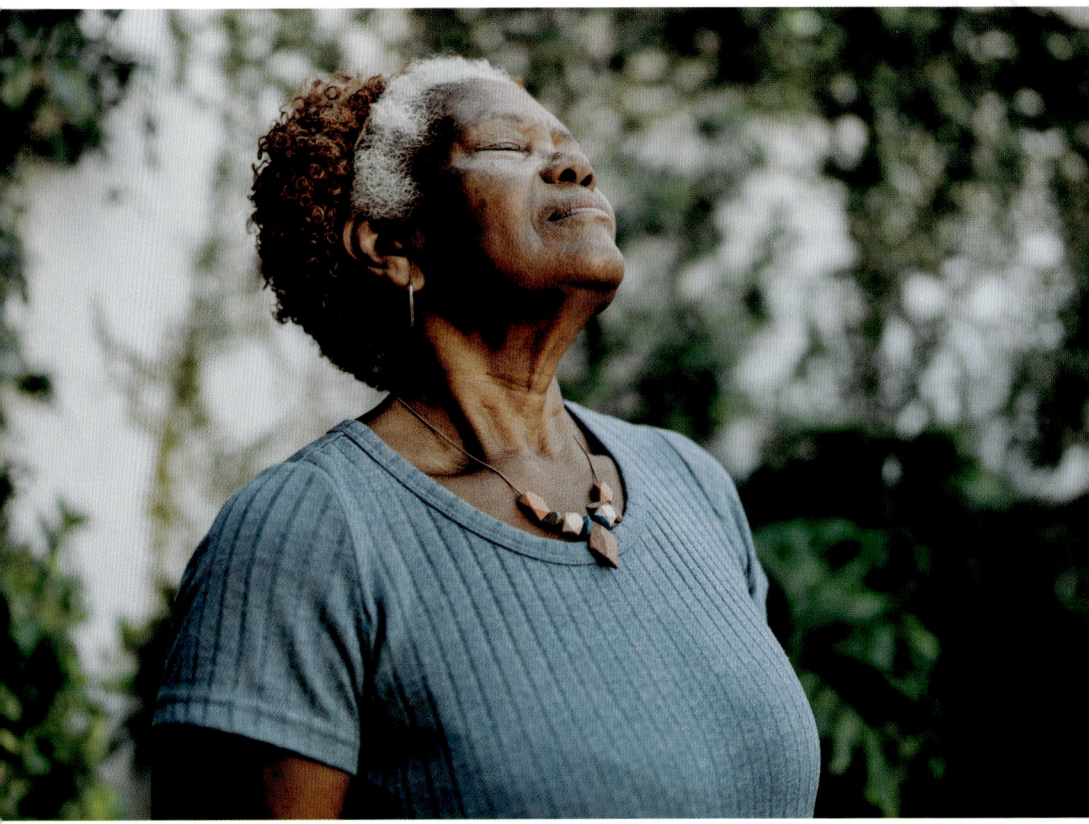

RELAXATION

While performing the exercises, try to remain relaxed, stay aware and recognise any tightness or tension that occurs in your body. Shoulders can rise up around the ears without you even realising it, fists can become clenched and jaws locked. Try to perform the exercises smoothly and gently, allowing them to flow. Once you're familiar with the movements, this will become easier. Dealing with any tensions in the body means that, eventually, they will disappear, making it easier to execute the movements required. When you fully relax, you will be slowing your heart rate down as well, and this can relieve stress. If you have high blood pressure, for example, it will be beneficial to learn to fully relax. Learning to relax can also improve your sleep. There is a separate chapter on relaxation and sleep on page 171.

CHAPTER 4

PREPARING FOR YOUR CHAIR PRACTICE

Before you begin your chair practice, here are some practical tips that will help you get the most out of your session.

HOW TO SIT

We all know how to sit and possibly this is something we all do too often, so these instructions may appear obvious. In order to get the most out of the seated exercises in this book, it's important to find yourself a comfortable chair, ideally without arms. This is because you'll move your arms and torso around and you need the space and freedom to do so. You don't want to be inhibited in any way. Also, make sure your chair is sturdy — folding chairs are fine but be aware that they have a habit of doing just that, folding. And it goes without saying that a chair on wheels is probably not a good idea. Please ensure your chair is solid, safe and comfortable.

Once seated on your chair, sit slightly away from the back so you're not leaning (unless instructed to do so in the exercise) or slouching, place your feet hip-width apart, knees placed over your ankles, and sit up as tall as you can, lengthening through your spine. Visualise helium balloons secured to the top of your head lifting you up and allowing you to grow taller as you sit.

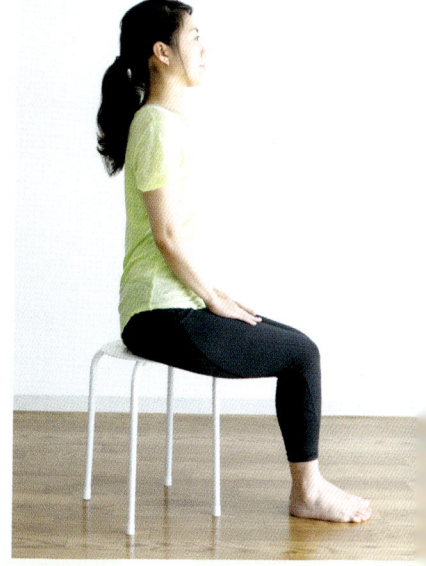

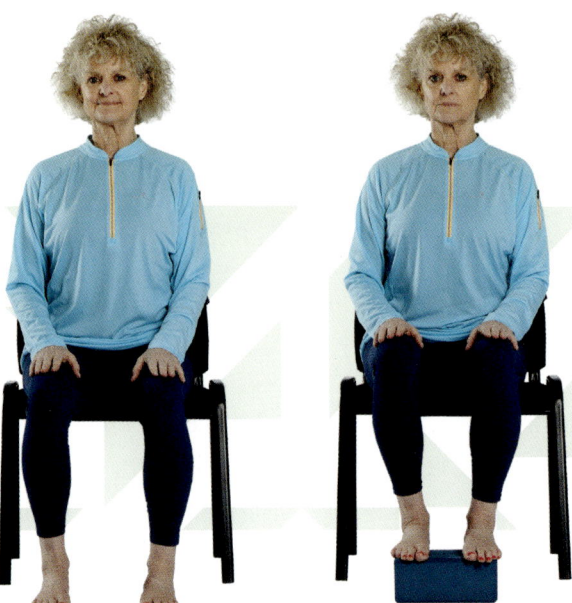

Once in this position, gently tilt your pelvis back and forth to find your neutral spine (*see* p. 23).

Rest your hands, palms down, on your thighs — it's always a good idea to take a moment to notice how you feel before you start the exercises. I'll take you through a body scan routine later, on page 43.

If you find that you're unable to sit with your legs at 90 degrees, then place a book or two or a yoga block under your feet to raise them up slightly so that they are at right angles.

STAYING HYDRATED

Have some water nearby. Especially in hot weather, it's important to keep hydrated as you'll lose fluid if you sweat. According to a report by the National Heart, Lung and Blood Institute, good hydration is linked to healthy ageing. Becoming dehydrated can increase the chance of urinary tract infections, can cause brain fog and dizziness and, yes, you've guessed it, it can increase the chance of falls. So keeping hydrated is important for us as we age, not only when we're exercising but throughout the day. If you don't like drinking plain water, flavour it with a slice of lemon or cucumber.

SAFETY TIPS

Make sure you have adequate space around your chair. You'll be moving your arms out to the side, and your legs will need space to extend in front of your chair and to the side — watch out for furniture like a low coffee table that can go unnoticed until you move. Always make sure you are comfortable with the exercises and that you understand the explanations given. If you experience any pain or niggles, stop; nothing should hurt. Yes, it might take effort and your muscles and joints might let you know that they're working hard, but there should be no real discomfort. If you're not sure whether or not the exercises are safe for you to do, please check with a health professional before beginning any of the routines.

Wear comfortable clothing for freedom of movement and ideally remain barefoot, as you'll benefit more from the feet exercises if your feet and toes can move freely and feel the ground beneath them.

THE IMPORTANCE OF ROUTINE

To get the most out of the exercises in this book, make an appointment with yourself to turn up regularly and get going. Maybe every morning or every other morning, a 10-minute routine, or more. None of this takes long, and if you're busy, it won't eat into your time, but it will make you feel better and more energised to face your day. At the back of the book, to start you off, you'll find some suggested routines.

MUSIC AND EXERCISE

According to the National Center for Health Research, music can make for a more enjoyable workout. It can improve the experience and even be motivational, adding an element of fun. Play your favourite tunes and lift those legs and arms to the beat!

If you choose to try the more dynamic 'cardio' workout in chapter 19, (see p.156) having a strong musical beat will provide the impetus to move faster. You'll have to work out the right tempo that suits your own personal timings, so experiment with different music.

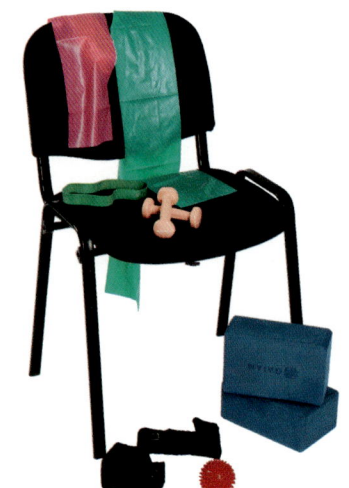

OPTIONAL EQUIPMENT

Light hand weights, cans of beans or small bottles of water can be used to add resistance when working your arms. If you choose to use these extras, please take care that they don't slip out of your hands. I suggest starting with 0.5kg or 1kg weights for your arms or legs unless you're already used to lifting weights, in which case, go with whatever weight you're used to. I've already mentioned improving muscle mass, and these will just add an extra element to your workout and go some way towards improving your strength even more. The same applies to ankle weights – you can fasten them around your ankles for all the leg exercises, if you so choose.

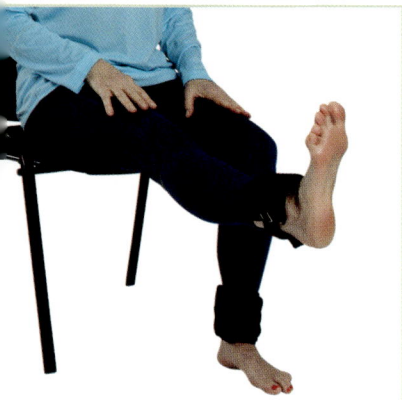

A resistance band is also a useful, versatile piece of kit to have, providing a different sort of workout. This will tone, strengthen and stretch those muscles, improving flexibility and mobility. Chapter 18 (*see* p. 141) will give you a full-body resistance band workout while seated. Resistance bands are easy to come by and they're not expensive. There are different sorts of resistance bands on the market: some are flat and some are tubular and others even have handles. I recommend the flatter band, which is what I use and you can see in the images. They come in different colours that indicate the resistance (strength) level. If you have joint pain, I suggest that you buy the lightest resistance band and see how you get on with it before advancing to a heavier resistance. There are also smaller round bands on the market that are useful and that I give you the option of using in the resistance band chapter.

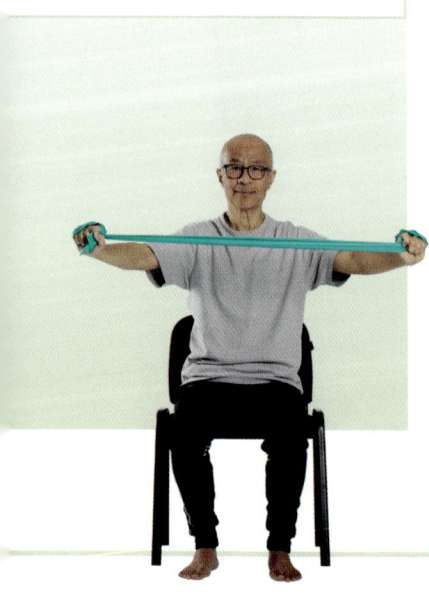

A tennis ball, foot roller or spikey ball can be used for massaging the feet, and this is something you can do when sitting on the sofa watching the TV.

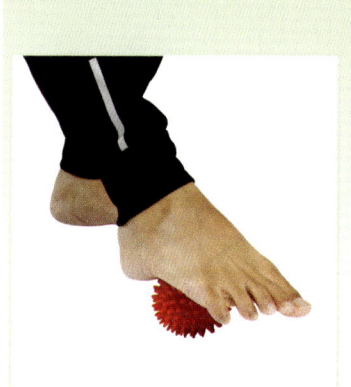

BREAST SURGERY

After breast surgery, arm and shoulder movement can be restricted and sometimes a tightness is felt in the armpit and chest. Practising the seated exercises in this book, especially the arm and shoulder exercises, can help you regain movement so that you can return quickly and comfortably back to your normal daily activities. Radiation can also affect arm and shoulder movement – so the same applies. Start slowly with the gentler beginners' exercises (marked 'B'), listen to your body, work within a comfortable range and then increase repetitions and move on to other exercises (marked 'I' for intermediate) when you're ready. Remember to take advice from your doctor, who will tell you when you can start exercising again and what is advisable to do.

ARTHRITIS

The exercises in this book are all low impact and therefore ideal for anyone suffering from this condition. In addition, they are gentle and help reduce pain, increasing the range of movement in stiff joints while improving strength and flexibility. It may be the last thing you feel like doing, but I promise you once you get going, you'll find yourself feeling so much better and more able. The charity Versus Arthritis has lots of information on exercise.

HIP REPLACEMENT

Chair Pilates and Yoga is an excellent way to strengthen and recover after a hip replacement.

A NOTE ON GENERAL MEDICAL AND MUSCULOSKELETAL PROBLEMS: If you've had hip, knee or breast surgery, or suffer from osteoporosis (neck or spine), serious back problems, arthritis or any other conditions that might have prevented you from exercising in the past, please take medical advice from a health professional before starting, just to make sure that you remain safe and that some of the moves aren't contraindicated as a result of your condition.

The exercises can restore your natural range of movement and improve your posture. Pre-operatively your postural alignment might have been altered due to pain or restricted movement. All this can be rectified and correct movement patterns and strength restored. Your physiotherapist will be able to advise you on when you can begin practising the exercises in this book and which movements are safe for you to perform.

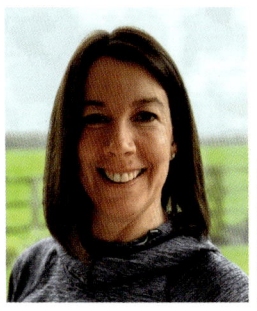

PROFESSIONAL ADVICE

SARA CARTER
PHYSIOTHERAPIST

Sara who works with older adults says:

'Movement is really important following hip replacement and in most circumstances people will be encouraged to be up and walking within a few days. Some movements may be limited, but this will vary based on the type of surgery and guidance given by the surgeon. Movement restrictions may include not bending the hip joint beyond 90 degrees, not crossing legs and not twisting at the hip. Chair Pilates and Yoga can be easily adapted to avoid these movements, for example doing the exercises from a higher chair to avoid excessive bending at the hip.

It is very normal to feel tired immediately following surgery; this is a big operation and the muscles and tissues around the hip will take time to heal. Chair-based Pilates and yoga is a really good way to begin strengthening the muscles while managing fatigue and any post-operative pain.

Sit to stand [*see* p. 127] is an exercise that is key to strengthening the glute muscles and, as rehab progresses, chair-based exercise can encourage control and balance. Sit to stand is one of the few dynamic exercises that is a bilateral support task, i.e. both feet are on the ground. It is easy to start compensating and avoiding using the operated hip; frequent practice and intentional sit-to-stand exercise helps ensure that the muscles on the operated side strengthen and you return to a normal movement pattern.'

KNEE REPLACEMENT

By practising Chair Pilates and Yoga, you will go some way to improving the strength of the muscles surrounding your knee, particularly the thigh muscles, and this will help you regain full range of movement to your knee. Pre-operatively you might have been limping and/or in pain and your movement limited, so give your body time to readjust. The balance, core strengthening and foot and ankle mobility exercises will all help you get back to normal. Your physiotherapist will be able to advise you on when you can begin practising the exercises in this book and which movements are safe for you to perform.

On knee replacement Sara says:

'A total knee replacement is usually done for severe arthritis and primarily used to eradicate the pain. The surgery involved in total knee replacement stretches the muscles around the knee resulting in bruising, swelling and weakness, so it is very important to start your exercises early to manage this.

There are two key elements to focus on in your rehab, the first being strengthening the muscles surrounding the knee. The two main muscle groups are the quadriceps on the front side of the knee and the hamstrings on the back side. Both these muscles cross the knee joint, therefore the stronger they are, the more protected the knee is. These will be targeted with exercises such as sit to stand and stand to sit [see p. 127].

The second is regaining the range of movement in the knee. The knee is a hinge joint, and the two main movements are flexion (bending) and extension (straightening). Chair-based exercises can be an excellent choice to incorporate into your rehab programme and can also be used to monitor progress, for example being able to bend the knee further during any knee flexion exercises.

As with any activity, it is important to listen to your body. Some pain may persist for a further few weeks/months and you should use this as a guide when participating in new activities. A moderate ache that settles quickly is normally acceptable; severe pain that takes hours to settle is not. Any concerns should be discussed with your GP or surgeon.'

CHAPTER 5

THE CHAIR EXERCISES

A gentle warm-up is always advised and should be performed before continuing with any general exercises, especially if you haven't done anything for a long time. I suggest starting with a body scan (p. 43), some gentle breathing (pp. 28–9), arm stretches (p. 61) and the roll down (p. 46). In addition, you might like to add in some neck mobility (p. 49) and spinal mobility (p. 57), if you feel particularly stiff in those areas, before continuing with anything else. Both the neck and spine have separate stand-alone chapters.

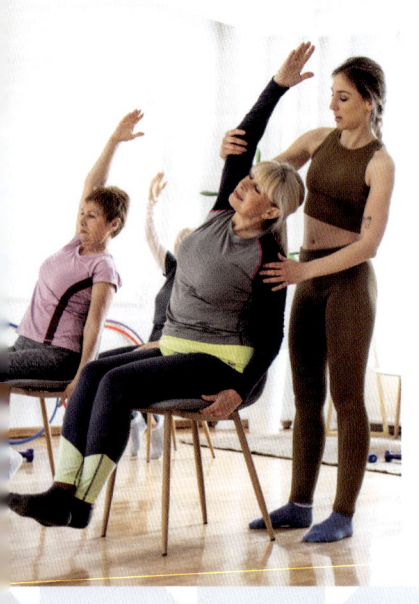

After this, we'll start by focusing on the upper body and then move to the lower body, but you can easily mix and match the exercises depending on your preferences. Maybe pick two arm exercises and two leg exercises, a couple of stretches and so forth. Or use one of the ready-made routines on pages 185 and 186. Or even just open the book randomly and have a go at whatever pops up.

You'll see that some exercises are marked with a **(B)** for beginners — if that is you, or you're nervous about exercising, or recovering from injury or illness, then stick to those simple movements to begin with. When you feel more confident, try some of the others, marked **(I)** for intermediate. And remember the number of repetitions that I suggest are just that: suggestions. You may feel like doing only a couple or you may feel like doing loads more. It's up to you.

BREATHING AND BODY SCAN (B)

Benefits

Some deep breathing, to begin with, will get you in the mood, help you to relax and start to connect you with your body by tuning in to how you feel.

Method

- Sit up tall on your chair, lengthen through the spine with your feet on the floor below your knees.
- Rest your hands on your thighs, either palms up or down, and try to keep your arms and shoulders relaxed.
- Maybe close your eyes for a moment (after you've read the instructions, obviously!).
- Begin by taking a gentle breath in through the nose – feel your ribcage expand as you do so.
- Breathe out through the mouth with a gentle sighing sound.
- Focus on your breath: feel the air enter your body through your nostrils and travel down into the lungs as your belly rises, before releasing, once again, out of your mouth.
- Complete 4 rounds, or more, if you're comfortable doing so. Take your time and enjoy the feeling that mindful breathing can create.

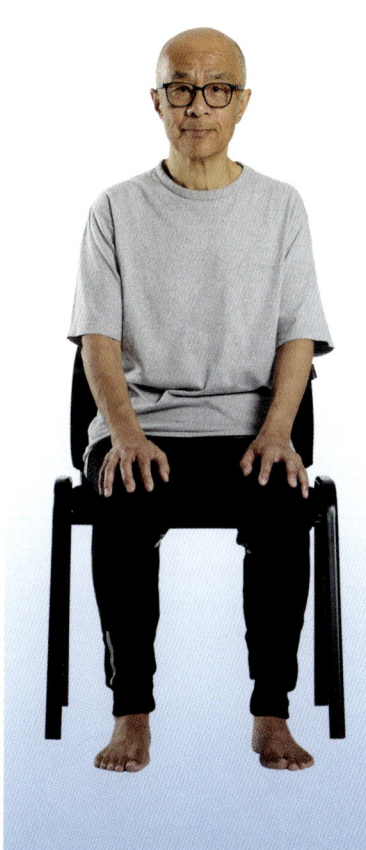

Once you've completed the breathing exercise, take a minute to perform a body scan.

- Think about how you feel physically. Are you tense? Relaxed? Are your shoulders up around your ears? Do you have any niggles or stiffness? Are you hot or cold?
- Just take a moment to notice what's going on in your body, maybe close your eyes for a time in order to focus more fully.
- If you do sense some discomfort, an ache, or a twinge of some sort, breathe in and as you do so, allow your attention to focus on the area of discomfort.
- Breathe out and let that discomfort go.
- If this feels odd, try it a few times and see what you observe; experiment.

It's a great way to start, as it helps you to become centred and prepares you for the exercises.

WAKE-UP STRETCHES (B)

Now we're going to stretch our arms in the air above our heads, allowing all tension to leave the body as we do so.

Benefits

By stretching your arms above your head (or to wherever you can), you will improve the flexibility and mobility of your shoulders and strengthen your arms. The movement also lengthens your spine and releases tension in your upper back. This stretch always feels good, which is why we sometimes automatically do it first thing in the morning when we wake up.

NOTE: If you can't lift your arms very high, or your shoulders are uncomfortable and stiff, then just raise your arms to wherever you feel you can. If one side of your body works better than the other side, the same applies: move to wherever you feel able as long as it's comfortable. Don't force anything.

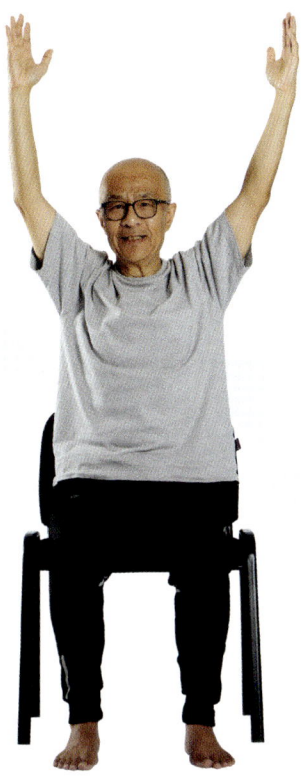 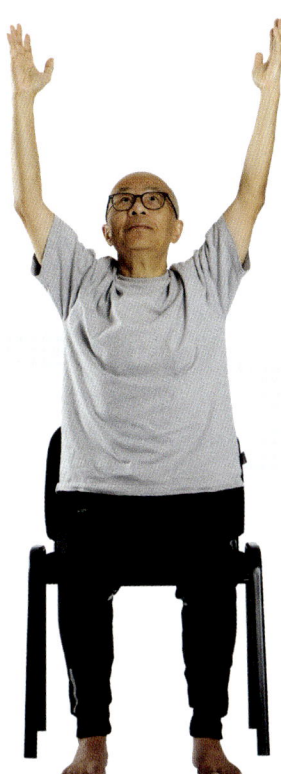

Method

- Sit up tall on your chair with a neutral spine (*see* p. 23). Breathe in.
- As you breathe out, lift both your arms out to the side of your body and let them float up above your head, as if they're being lifted up on a cloud, forming a gentle stretch.
- Lengthen your fingers to the ceiling and, as long as your neck is comfortable, look up towards your hands.
- Breathe in again with your arms still lengthened above your head (or wherever they reach).
- As you breathe out, gently push the air from of your lungs with a big sigh as you return your head and arms to the start position.
- Try to be conscious of your breath (return to page 28 if you need reminding about the importance of breathing). Mindful breathing will help you perform the exercise comfortably and is a good way to prepare your body for more exercise.

ROLL DOWN (B)

In a general mat Pilates class, we stand tall and roll down like a rag doll, and in yoga too there is a forward bend pose. Both of these are excellent stretches for your lower back and hamstrings (back of your thighs), and you can perform this adapted version perfectly well while seated.

If you suffer from back problems only move your torso to wherever it feels comfortable; don't force anything and if you can only bend or move a little way, that's fine.

Benefits

This forward movement can relieve back stiffness, as it improves spinal mobility and allows the spinal discs to expand. It also helps develop that much-needed flexibility for freedom of movement in everyday life, like bending (think gardening, picking something up off the floor or putting your shoes on).

NOTE: If putting your head down makes you feel dizzy, then either omit this exercise or when you uncurl your spine back to a sitting position, take it very, very slowly and try not to hold your breath.

You'll see that I mention breathing all the time throughout the book because it's so easy to forget to breathe properly when exercising, but you'll find if you do breathe, then the movements will feel easier and more comfortable.

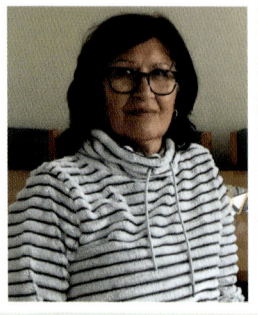

CASE STUDY

EMMA BARBER
AGE 72

'Chair Pilates and Yoga is exactly what you need to be doing all the time; it's so very helpful. Exercise has really cured my bad back; it has been of great benefit. If I don't do it, and particularly the roll down, my back stiffens.'

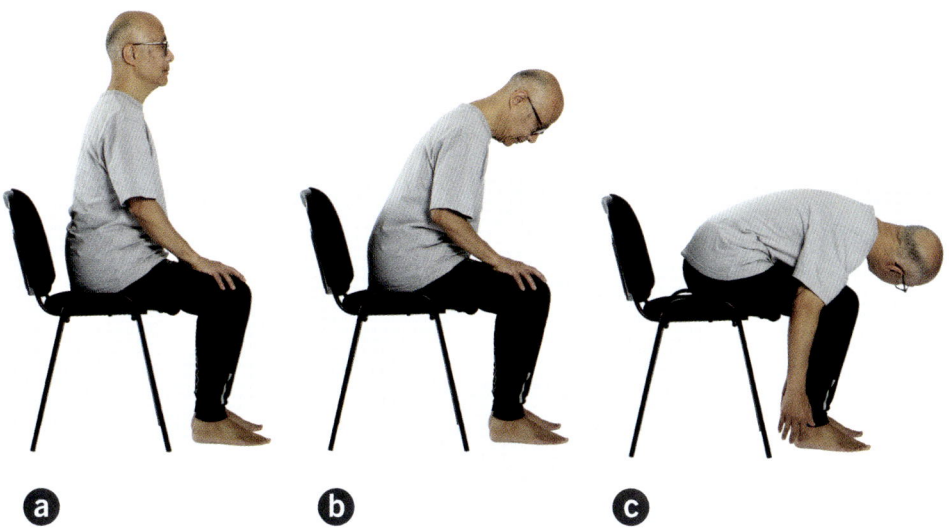

Method

- Sit up tall on your chair and keep your shoulders relaxed.
- Allow your arms to hang by your sides or rest on your thighs for support and engage your abdominal muscles. **a**
- Take a breath in and feel your rib cage expand as you do so.
- As you breathe out through your mouth, bring your chin gently down on to your chest.
- Slowly begin to roll yourself down towards your thighs and between your knees. **b**
- Stop when you come to a comfortable point of tension.
- Once you reach that place of tension, allow your arms to hang loose from your shoulders on either side of your legs like a rag doll – you might even be able to touch the floor with your fingertips. **c**
- Your neck should be relaxed and your head heavy as you hang there. Maybe rock your head gently back and forth to release any tension that might be present in your neck.
- Breathe naturally as you hold this position for a silent, slow count of four.
- Take a breath in again, into your ribcage, with your abdominal muscles still engaged.

- As you breathe out, start to uncurl your body back up to a sitting position, vertebra by vertebra, slowly building your spine, strong and straight and tall.
- As you reach the top, keep your chin on your chest until the very last second, then uncurl lengthening through the neck back to a sitting position and imagine helium balloons lifting you up as you grow taller.
- Take a moment here at the top.
- Breathe in again and this time pull up your pelvic floor muscles (*see* p. 26) and try to keep them engaged throughout the next repetition.
- Repeat the roll down several more times. You might find that you can go lower each time as your spine warms up.

Remember this is not a competition. Just roll down to wherever it feels comfortable for you. It may be a little way or all the way so that your fingers reach the floor, it doesn't matter; you will still be mobilising and stretching your spine.

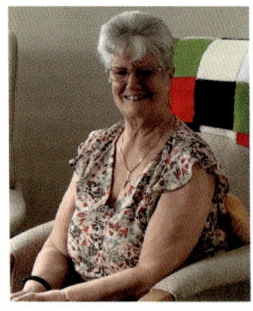

CASE STUDY

GLENNIS ROLFE
AGE 78

'Chair Pilates and Yoga helps you to keep up keeping fit – even if you can only manage to exercise one joint or muscle or limb, do it and try two next time and so on. Don't get disheartened, keep at it. Some days it's easier than other days. Due to being knocked down by a car I have problems now with my legs, shoulders, neck and hips. I have an artificial knee joint too. But I love my independence and don't want to lose it, so seated exercise really helps me to maintain that.'

CHAPTER 6

THE NECK

Ageing can cause wear and tear in our necks and our discs and joints can slowly degenerate. Cervical spondylosis is extremely common. More than 85 per cent of people over the age of 60 are affected.

Gently stretching any weakened neck muscles is beneficial. A stiff neck and achy muscles in the upper back can sometimes be caused by sleeping in an awkward position, sitting at a desk all day or just general bad posture, and this can, for some, trigger a headache. Perform these exercises smoothly and listen to your body. If your neck feels too uncomfortable at any point, stop. If you do have a stiff neck, then these exercises will relieve some of the discomfort, although moving it may feel counterintuitive.

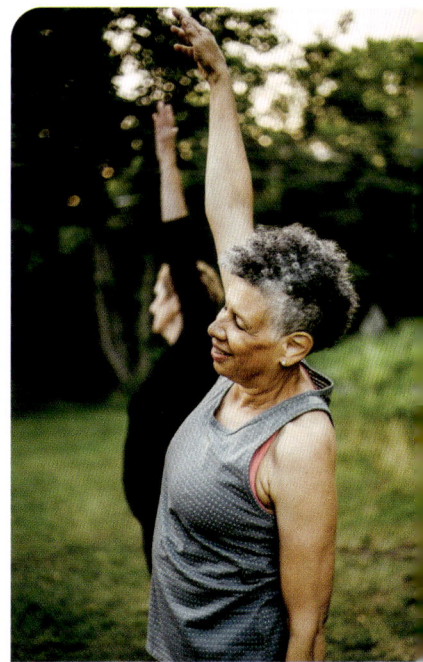

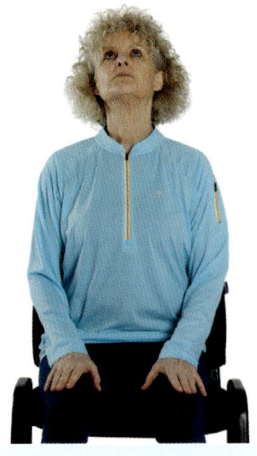
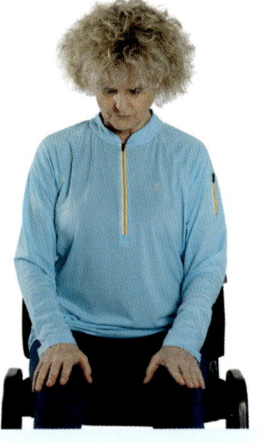
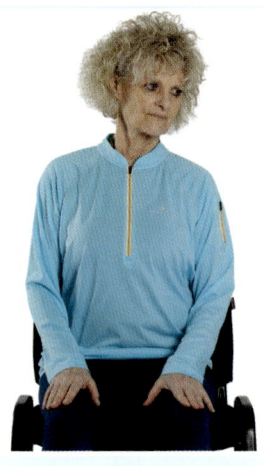

NUMBERS (B)

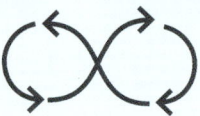

Benefits

This first exercise, Numbers, is a fun and gentle way to start mobilising your neck before the stretch exercise that follows. It will also improve your coordination.

Method

- Sit up tall on your chair, lengthen through the spine with your feet on the floor below your knees.
- Imagine those helium balloons attached to the top of your head, lifting you upwards; feel how your spine lengthens as you visualise this image.
- Fix your gaze on something ahead of you – this will help you focus on the movement. Or if you prefer, close your eyes.
- Keep your shoulders relaxed and your chin raised.
- Breathing normally, draw a circle with your nose, taking your neck with you.
- Do this a couple of times one way.
- Reverse the rotation the other way.
- Now choose a number – eight is a good one to start with – and draw the number eight with your nose, taking your head and neck with you. Keep the movement small and smooth.
- Follow this with the number two and then try the number four – and don't forget to reverse the movement!

SIDE NECK STRETCHES (B)

Benefits

This is a simple tilt of the head to the side towards your shoulder; it may be a tiny movement for you or much bigger depending on the flexibility of your neck, just do what's right for you and keep it comfortable. Whatever you choose to do will benefit those stiff neck muscles.

NOTE: You might find that one side of your neck is more flexible than the other, so on the stiffer side, consider holding the stretch for a little longer, but don't forget to breathe.

Method

- Sit up tall on your chair with a neutral spine.
- Take a breath in through the nose and out through the mouth before you move, to allow any tension to release; if your neck is particularly stiff, then take a few more breaths before you stretch your neck to the side.
- As you breathe out, visualise letting go of the tension in your neck.
- When you're ready, breathe in again.
- As you breathe out, tilt your right ear towards your right shoulder, gently stretching out the opposite side of your neck and upper back muscles.
- Breathe normally as you hold the stretch for a silent count of four.
- Breathe in again and as you breathe out, raise your head back up to centre and sit up tall.
- Perform the exercise on both sides 4 times.

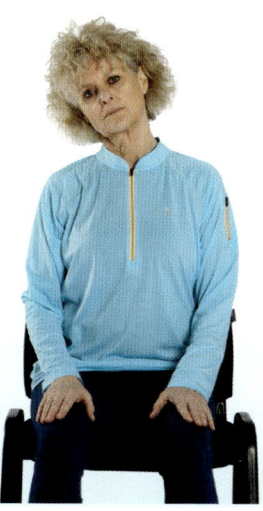 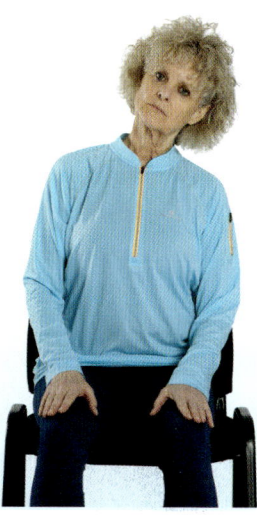

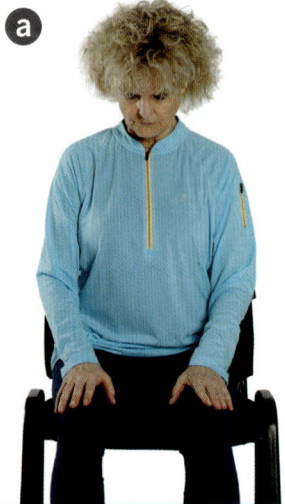

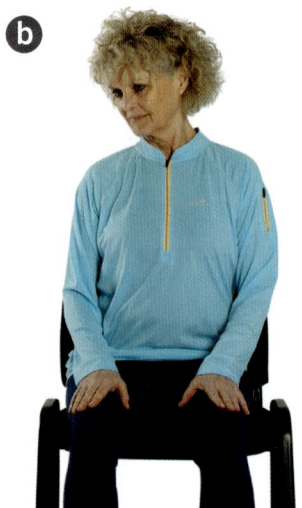

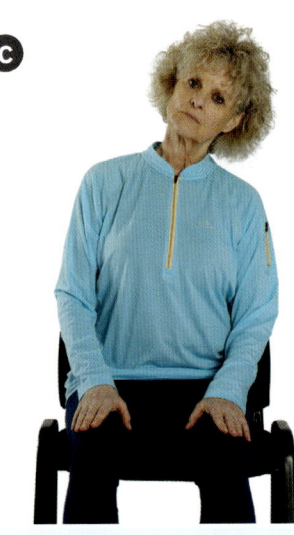

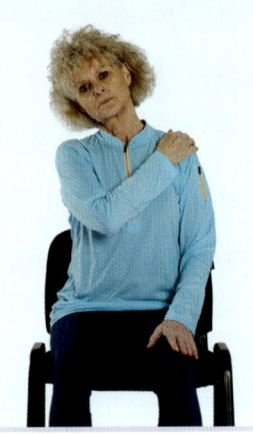

NOTE: If you find that your shoulder rises up as you drop your ear to your opposite shoulder, place a hand on it to encourage it to stay put.

- After completing the repetitions for the side neck stretch exercise, sit upright and tall again.
- Breathe in and drop your chin down on to your chest as you breathe out.
- Gently rotate your neck to one side, again tilting your ear towards your shoulder, but don't take your head beyond your shoulder.
- Breathe in again as you hold the stretch for the count of four.
- As you breathe out, drop your chin back down towards your chest.
- Breathe in and when you breathe out roll to the other shoulder, tilting your left ear towards it.
- Gently rotate from side to side, letting the weight of your head carry it slowly down to your chest and then over to the other side.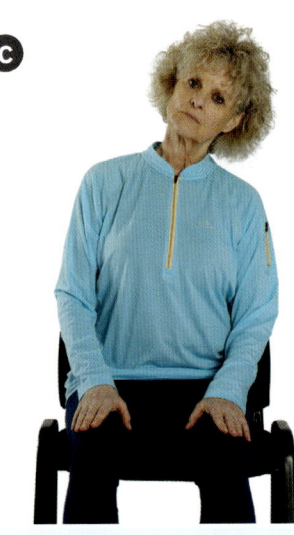
- Repeat twice on either side if you're comfortable doing so, then return to centre and lift up your head, lengthening through your neck and spine once again.

HEAD TURNS (B)

Benefits

This exercise is a great neck loosener — perfect for a stiff neck. However, if your neck is very stiff or sore, just move it a little way and don't force it.

Method

- Sit up tall on your chair.
- Take a breath in and as you breathe out turn your head to your right as if you're looking for something over your shoulder.
- Hold the position as you breathe in again, then as you breathe out move your head back and face forwards.
- Breathe in as you face front and as you breathe out turn your head to the left.
- Repeat 4 times or more.

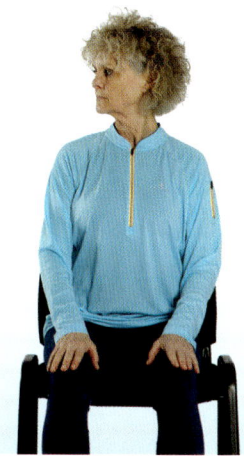

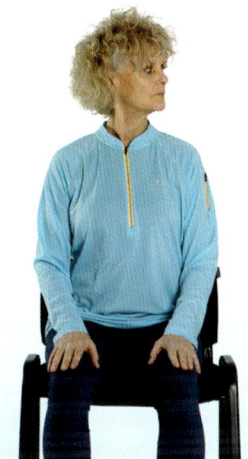

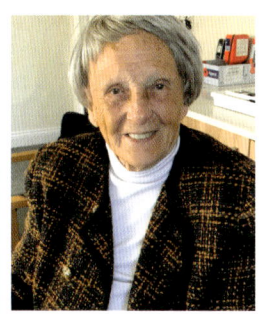

CASE STUDY

BRIDGET WHITE
AGE 95

'I need to do the neck exercises so that I can continue to look over my shoulder when I'm out and about on my mobility scooter, to keep safe. As I don't walk now, the flexing and pointing of the feet and rotating of the ankles is good to do as are the shoulder exercises — I injured my shoulder and the shoulder exercises have helped to give it more movement. Chair Pilates and Yoga is good fun and I do my best. I mustn't give in — it's all in the mind — and I do have a tiresomely cheerful disposition, which helps!'

CHAPTER 7

SHOULDERS

If you have problems with your shoulders, take this section slowly; perform fewer rotations if anything feels uncomfortable. Revisit this chapter as many times as you like. It's simple and can relax tired or tense shoulders and takes no time at all.

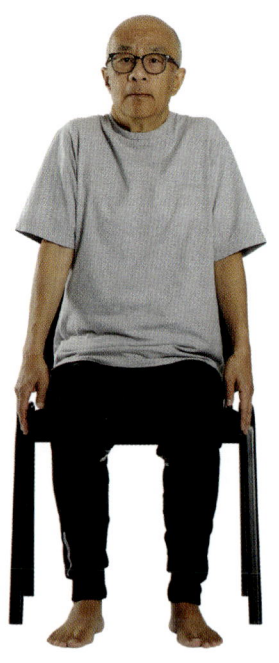

SHOULDER ROLLS (B)

Benefits

We can carry a lot of tension in our shoulders and so doing these simple rotations can be a welcome way to release tightness in this area. If you have specific problems with your shoulders, like a frozen shoulder or shoulder impingement, for example, take advice from your health professional about the suitability of these exercises for you.

Method

- Sit up tall on your chair with a neutral spine and breathe normally.

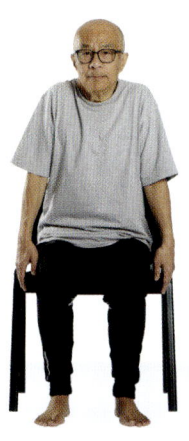

- Gently raise both your shoulders upwards towards your ears.
- Slowly rotate them forwards 4 times.
- Now rotate your shoulders gently backwards 4 times.
- If you feel that your shoulders could benefit from more rotations, then repeat the exercise.

SHOULDER AND CHEST OPENER (B)

Benefits

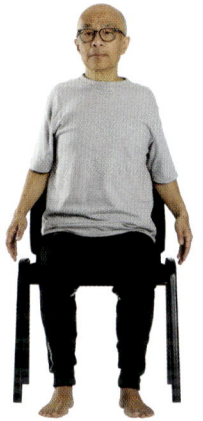

This shoulder exercise has the added benefit of stretching out your pectoral muscles (chest muscles), which can become very tight. It will also go some way towards improving your posture if you tend to be hunched, as well as relieving any tension in your shoulders.

Method

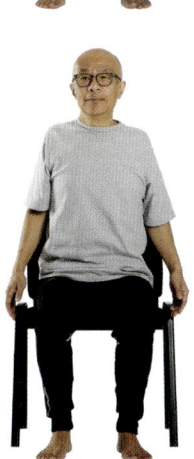

- Sit up tall on your chair.
- Gently raise both your shoulders up towards your ears and move them backwards so that you feel your chest opening out as you do so.
- Slide your shoulder blades down your back towards the seat of your chair – this will stretch your chest even more.
- Hold for a beat before releasing.
- Repeat 4 times.

CASE STUDY

JOHN BROWN
AGE 68

'Having retired three years ago from my position as director of a catering business, which had been an active role, I was diagnosed with breast cancer. After a mastectomy, it was discovered that I had the early stages of Parkinson's disease. I was conscious that I needed to improve my level of fitness, but I was also aware that this exercise could not be too strenuous. I also needed to join an online course. I now attend Harri's Chair Pilates and Yoga classes via Zoom twice a week and that's been ideal. Now that I'm 68 years old, I have found the mix of gentle stretching, strength and mobility exercises are most suited to my circumstances.'

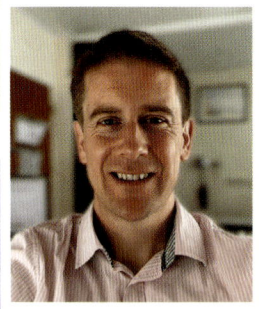

PROFESSIONAL ADVICE

DR MATTHEW ROBINSON
GENERAL PRACTITIONER

Matthew says:

'Parkinson's disease can bring with it a number of problems including poor balance [and] difficulties in walking and moving, as well as episodes of "freezing". Studies show that regular physical activity can benefit people with Parkinson's disease in a number of ways, including increasing walking distance and speed, reduced episodes of freezing, improved balance and better mental health. All of these benefits help to improve function and mobility, reduce falls and increase and prolong independence. The benefits start even before symptoms appear, so the sooner activity levels are increased, the better.'

CHAPTER 8

THE SPINE

Backache is a common ailment and can sadly become more debilitating as we age, so it pays to work on keeping the spine mobile and strong. The lower back is often where most people suffer discomfort, and you can read more about this and the other areas of the spine in more detail on page 22. But if you find you wake up every morning with a stiff lower back or your back aches after sitting at your desk for a prolonged period of time, the following exercises will help alleviate those niggles, stretch out the tight areas and help to keep the spine flexible and strong.

SPINAL UNDULATIONS (B)

Benefits

You may be familiar with the cat and cow postures in yoga. This exercise is a seated adaptation that will mobilise the spine and open out the chest a little further, stretching tight pectoral muscles (chest). If your posture has a tendency to be hunched or slouched and you are round-shouldered, your chest muscles can become tight. Also by opening out your chest in the second part of this exercise, your breathing can improve, giving those lungs more space to expand.

Beautiful young people are accidents of nature, but beautiful old people are works of art.'

Eleanor Roosevelt

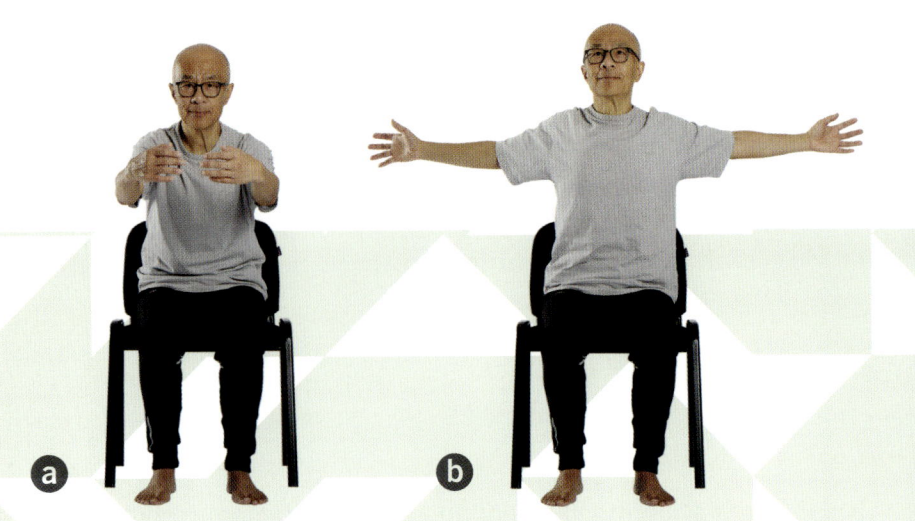

Method

- Sit up tall on your chair, lengthen through the spine with your feet parallel on the floor below your knees.
- Engage your abdominal muscles and/or your pelvic floor muscles.
- Breathe in, feeling your ribcage expand.
- As you breathe out round your arms in front of your chest as if you are hugging a tree or a big beach ball. **a**
- Hold this position for a moment, breathing normally for a silent count of four.
- Breathe in again and as you breathe out go the opposite way, opening out your arms to the sides of your body, as if you are greeting a long-lost friend. **b**
- Lean back slightly as you look up at the ceiling, feeling a good stretch across your chest.
- Hold this stretch, breathing normally, for a silent count of four.
- Breathe in again and as you breathe out, return to sitting upright.
- Repeat 4 times.
- If you prefer, you can make it a more dynamic movement – breathing in as you 'hug the tree', breathing out as you open your arms and stretch in the other direction.

SPINAL ROTATION (TWISTING) (B)

Benefits

This is an effective exercise that mobilises the spine in a gentle twisting motion. If you have back problems or are excessively stiff, only rotate as far as you are comfortable; don't force the movement.

Method

- Sit up tall on your chair.
- Take your right hand and hold your left forearm behind your wrist. **a**
- Rotate your left arm to take hold of your right forearm behind the wrist. Engage your abdominal muscles and/or your pelvic floor muscles.
- Take a breath in before you move and then breathe out as you rotate your torso to the right, taking your head and neck with you and looking over your shoulder. **b**
- Try to keep your shoulders relaxed as they might decide to shift upwards towards your ears.
- Breathe in as you hold the position for a moment and then breathe out as you return to facing forwards.
- Breathe in again and as you breathe out, rotate your torso to the left. **c**
- Breathe in as you hold and then as you breathe out return to the front.
- Repeat 4 times — you might find you can rotate a little bit further each time.

NOTE: If you have serious back problems, please take advice from your health professional about the suitability of rotational exercises.

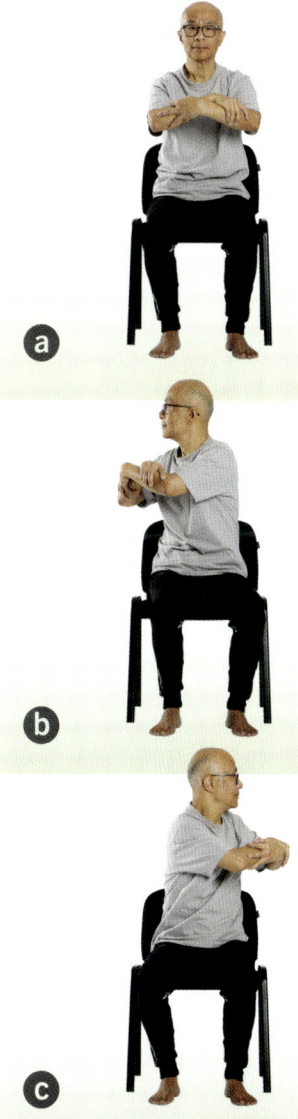

LATERAL FLEXION 1 (SIDE BENDING) (B)

Benefits

This exercise will lengthen and stretch the side of your torso improving your flexibility. Tight muscles along the side of your body can sometimes lead to shoulder and neck problems. Your lower back will also benefit from this stretch. Don't go too far and take care not to topple off the chair! This is a gentle sideways stretch that should feel comfortable and you shouldn't need to go far to feel it.

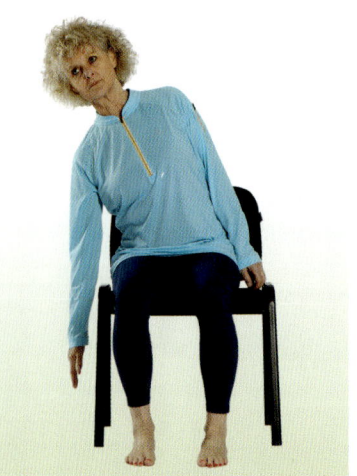

Method

- Sit up tall on your chair.
- Check that your shoulders are relaxed and let your arms hang by your sides.
- Take a breath in to prepare.
- Breathe out and slowly slide one hand down the side of your chair and lean gently towards it, lengthening your fingers as you do so, until you feel a stretch on the opposite side of your body.
- Breathe in again, make sure your abdominal muscles are engaged.
- As you breathe out return your torso to an upright position. Lengthen through your spine as you do so.
- Repeat on the other side.
- Repeat 4 times.

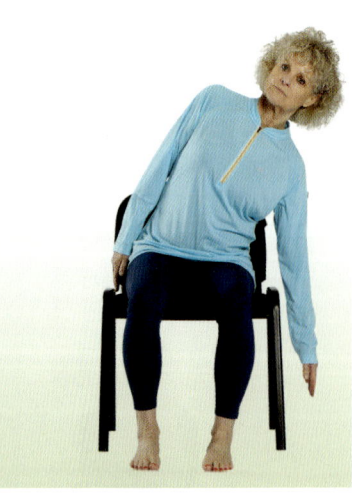

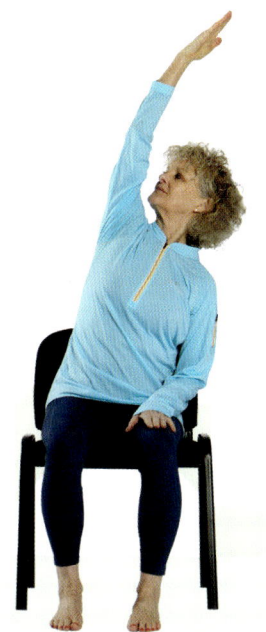 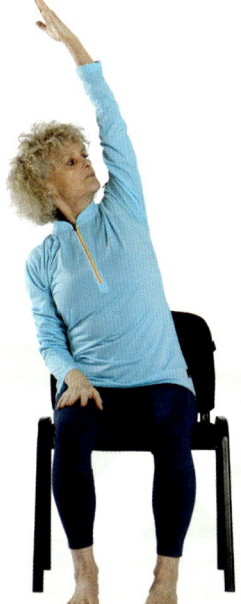

LATERAL FLEXION 2 (B)

Benefits

This exercise is an extension of the previous one. It has the added benefit of an arm stretch, which adds a greater lengthening to the side of your torso from your lower back to your shoulder.

Method

- Sit up tall on your chair.
- Breathe in and when you breathe out, lift your right arm up in the air and extend it over your head to the opposite side. Only stretch to a position you feel comfortable in.
- Hold for a beat, breathe in again and turn your head towards your arm if your neck allows.
- Breathe out and return your arm to centre above you; as you do so, stretch your arm and fingers upwards towards the ceiling.
- Return your arm to your side.
- Repeat with the other arm.
- Repeat 4 times.

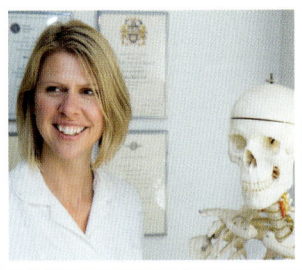

PROFESSIONAL ADVICE

JANE KAUSHAL
OSTEOPATH

Jane says:

'The reason why it is important to increase or maintain bone mass in older age is to prevent osteoporosis-related fractures. In order to prevent reduction in bone mass, it is helpful to overload the bones with jumping type activities or heavy weight training. Pilates or yoga practice would need to be very vigorous to 'tick these boxes'. However Chair Pilates and Yoga can have an even more important impact on the prevention of osteoporosis-related fractures because it provides significant benefits to balance, postural stability, muscle strength and flexibility. This all helps with fall prevention. While being more active improves health in numerous ways, it can mean that you are more likely to fall. This is not so likely to be the case if you regularly practise Chair Pilates and Yoga, even if the session is gentle.'

CHAPTER 9

HANDS, WRISTS, ELBOWS AND FINGERS

Our hands, wrists and fingers are probably not a part of our anatomy that we think of exercising very often, but as we age, and depending on our work, hobbies and genetics, they can become stiff and tender, and for some arthritis might be an issue, causing swelling, stiffness and deformity. Our hands, of course, are actually the first point of contact for many everyday activities — so keep them moving.

Strengthening and stretching your hands can improve their function and the blood flow to this part of your body. This is paramount to making sure you can still grip the handle of a mug (or a small hand weight, for some of these exercises), crochet, sew or knit, use a pen to write with and so much more. Our hands and fingers and wrists, like our feet, are so often taken for granted.

NOTE: If extending your arms out in front of your torso for any length of time is hard, then sit at a table and rest your forearms on the tabletop for the following exercises.

If you decide to do all the exercises in this section and you find that your shoulders become tense, just perform a few gentle shoulder rolls (*see* pp. 54–5) to relieve any tension that might have built up.

FOREARM PRONATION AND SUPINATION

Benefits

This is a very simple exercise for rotating the forearm, which is important for everyday activities like turning a doorknob or eating with a fork or spoon, among other things. Pronation is when the hand is facing downwards and supination is when the palm is facing upwards.

Method

- Sit up tall on your chair, lengthen through the spine with your feet parallel on the floor below your knees.
- Find your neutral spine (*see* p. 23) and breathe normally.
- Extend your arms out in front of you with a slight bend at the elbow, palms facing upwards (pronated). **a**
- Turn your hands and forearms the other way so that your palms are facing downwards (supinated). **b**
- Repeat 8 times back and forth.

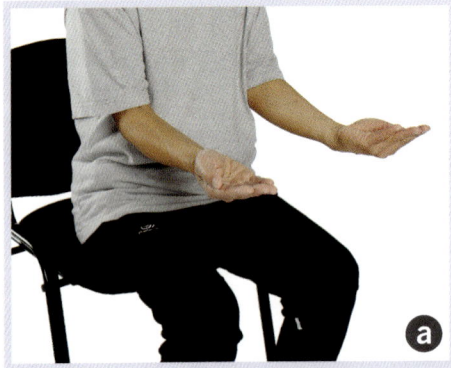
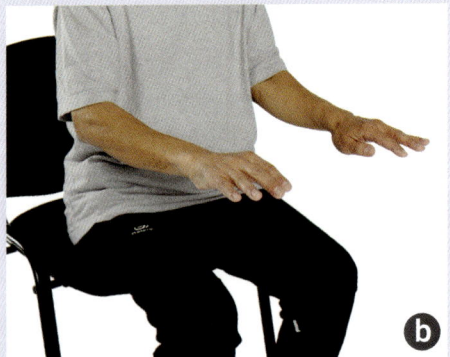

PIANO PLAYING FINGERS (B)

Benefits

This simple exercise will mobilise and strengthen your fingers. If you have stiff or arthritic fingers, then this exercise can go some way towards relieving any discomfort you might suffer from. If you do a lot of repetitive movements with your fingers, like crochet, stopping what you are doing, taking a break from the creative activity and 'playing the piano' can help to relieve finger aches.

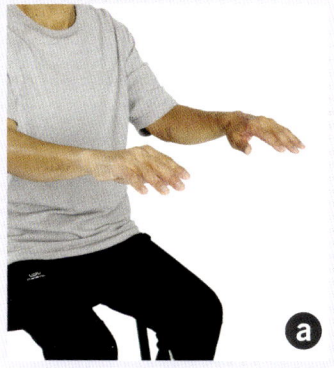

Method

- Sit up tall on your chair and breathe normally.
- Extend your arms out in front of you and spread your fingers as wide as they will go, then 'play the piano'. **a**
- If you like you can also move your arms so that they are outstretched from the sides of your body, like aeroplane wings, all the time playing the piano with your fingers. **b**
- Return your arms to centre.
- Repeat 4 times.

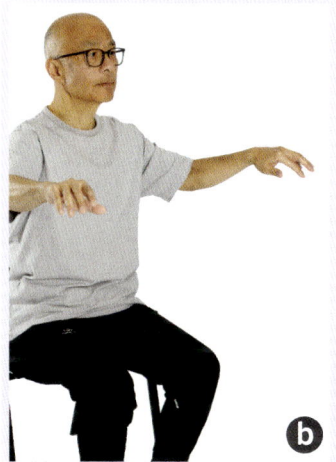

NOTE: A research study published in *The Lancet* in 2015 demonstrated that rheumatoid arthritis sufferers who performed daily hand exercises as part of their treatment found their hand function improved. Fingers became more flexible and their grip strengthened. Those in the study showed twice the improvement compared to those who didn't practise the exercises.

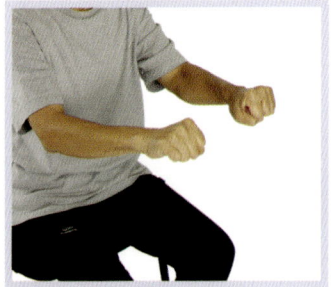

CURL AND STRETCH (B)

Benefits

This is another simple exercise for your hands, wrists and fingers, which mobilises, strengthens and improves flexibility.

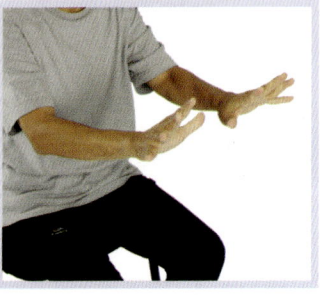

Method

- Sit up tall on your chair and breathe normally.
- Extend your arms out in front of you and form fists with your hands.
- Now spread your fingers out wide, stretching the palms of your hands and fingers.
- Alternate between clenched fist and open palm 8 times.
- For the next part of this routine, hold your right forearm with your left hand for support.
- Make a fist with your right hand then raise and lower your wrist 8 times.
- Repeat on the other side.
- Return to your right side, holding on to your forearm again with your left hand for support.
- Keeping your fingers relaxed, rotate your wrist 4 times one way and 4 times the other way.
- Repeat on the other side.
- Rest your arms and hands and rotate your shoulders if they feel tense.

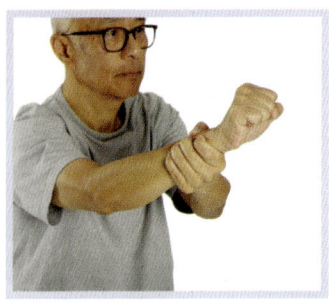

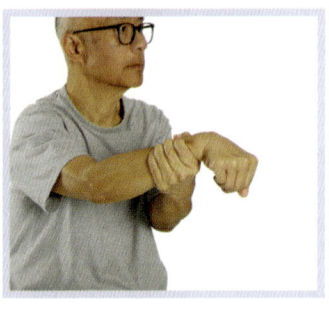

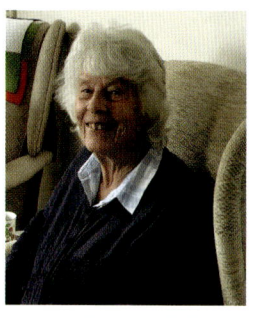

CASE STUDY

HELEN SMITH
AGE 86

'Gardening keeps me fit, so do my great-grandchildren, and I walk too. Chair Pilates and Yoga sessions are jolly good; it makes you do it, the exercise. I find it's also relaxing, and you can take the exercises home and repeat them.'

THUMBS UP (B)

Benefits

The following thumb stretch exercise will encourage normal movement and strengthen the muscles around the joint. If you suffer from osteoarthritis in the thumb joint, this might go some way to relieving the discomfort.

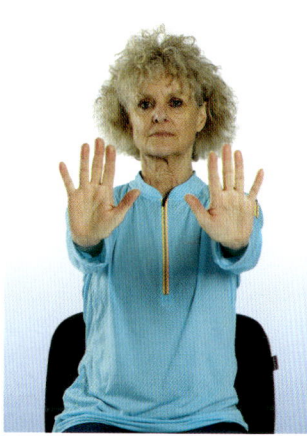

Method

- Extend your arms out in front of your torso as if you were stopping traffic.
- Move your thumbs across the palms of your hands so the tip of your thumb reaches the base of your little finger.
- Repeat 8 times.
- Now, for finer movements and coordination of your thumb, you're going to move the thumb to each finger. You'll bend each one in turn so that it meets the tip of your thumb.
- Start by touching the tip of your forefinger, then progress on to the middle finger, fourth finger, then little finger.
- When you've completed this, work backwards, from little finger to forefinger. You can perform this with one hand at a time or both at the same time.
- Repeat 4 times.

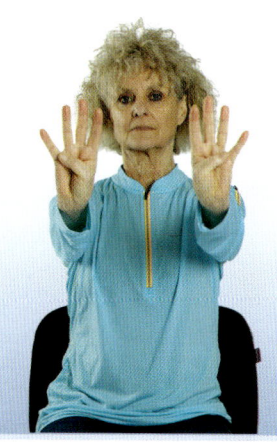

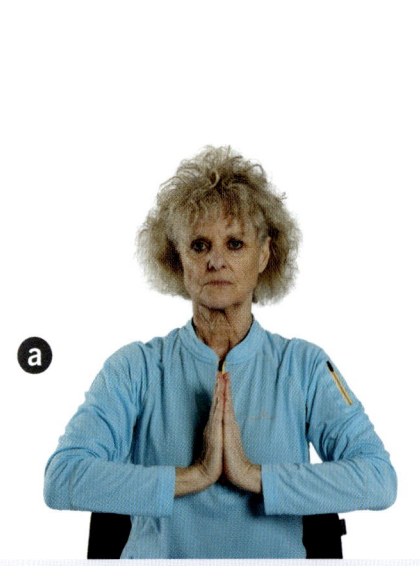

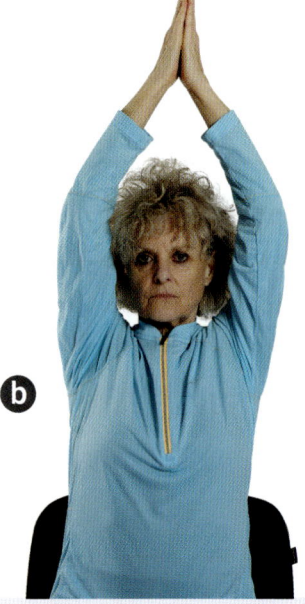

PALMS TOGETHER (B)

Benefits

Although this is a wrist exercise, as you raise your arms in the air above your head you will also be improving your shoulder strength and mobility. If you've attended yoga classes, you will recognise the hands placed in a prayer position with fingers lengthened as Anjali mudra, which is often used as a greeting in Asian countries. It's also a mark of acceptance and peace.

Method

- Sit up tall on your chair.
- Bring your hands together in the prayer position with your thumbs facing your chest and elbows out to the side.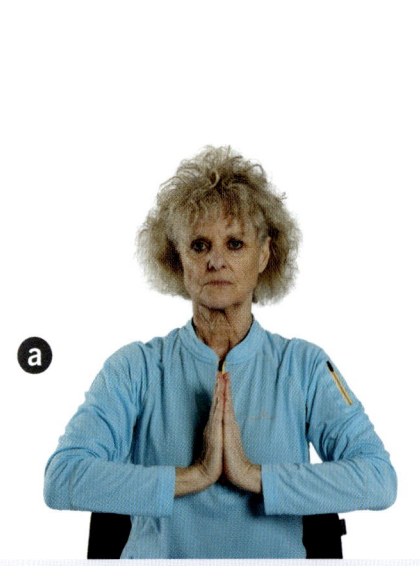
- Take a breath in and as you breathe out, keeping the palms of your hands glued together, raise your arms in the air above your head.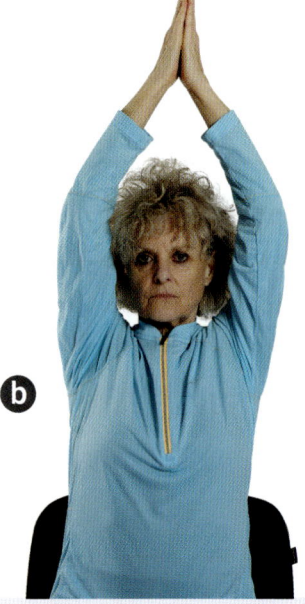
- Breathe in as you hold this position above your head for a beat.
- As you breathe out, with your hands still pressed together, lower your arms back down to the start position in front of your chest.
- Repeat 4 times.

CHAPTER 10

ARMS, SHOULDERS AND BACK

In this exercise section, you'll find lots of arm exercises to choose from, which you can mix and match depending on your preferences. Once again, I've marked the easier ones with a **(B)** for beginners and the more advanced ones with an **(I)** for intermediate. For a couple of general warm-up shoulder rotation exercises see pages 54–5.

If you wish to use light hand weights, please go ahead and do so. If you have a resistance band, there's a separate chapter (*see* p. 141) for a whole body workout using this piece of kit, including more arm, shoulder and back exercises.

The following exercises will strengthen your arms, shoulders and upper back, increase flexibility and improve coordination.

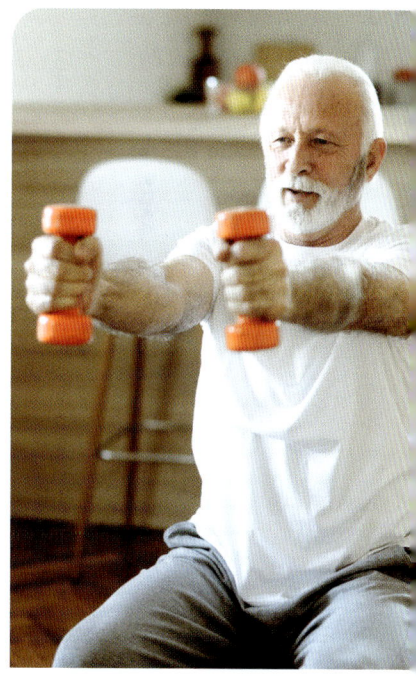

BICEPS (B)

These are the muscles at the front of your upper arm; they help bend the elbow and supinate the arm (rotate with your palm upwards). Before you start, decide whether you feel you'd like to use hand weights (or tins or small water bottles) for extra resistance. If you do, grab them now and have them ready. Beginners can omit these props.

Benefits

We use our bicep muscles for everything – from lifting up a mug of tea or coffee to turning a doorknob, picking things up or pulling something towards us. But like the rest of our body, we need to work on them to keep them functioning efficiently as we age and to maintain or improve muscle mass.

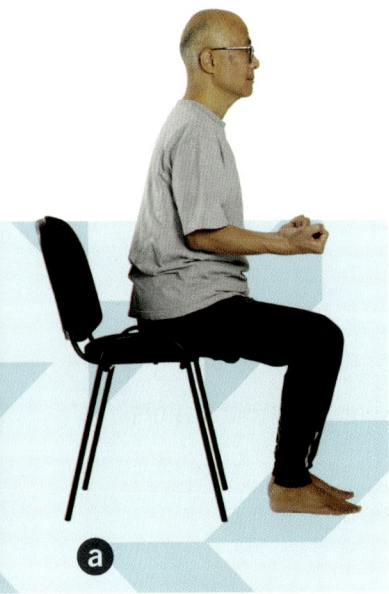

Method

- Sit up tall on your chair with your feet parallel on the floor below your knees.
- Bend your arms so that your elbows hug your ribcage and your forearms are out in front of you at right angles with your palms facing upwards.
- Gently make a fist with your hands if you're not using hand weights. **a**
- Breathe in as you lift your hands and forearms up to your shoulders, keeping your elbows squeezing your ribcage. **b**
- Breathe out as you lower your forearms back to the start position.
- Repeat 8 times.

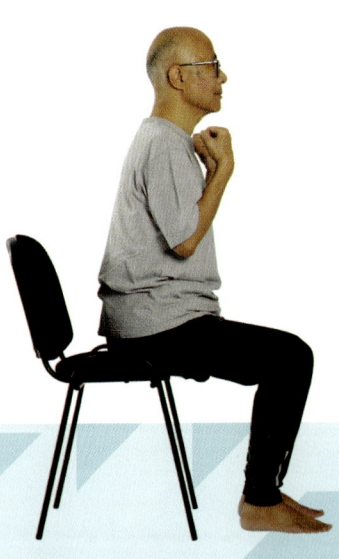

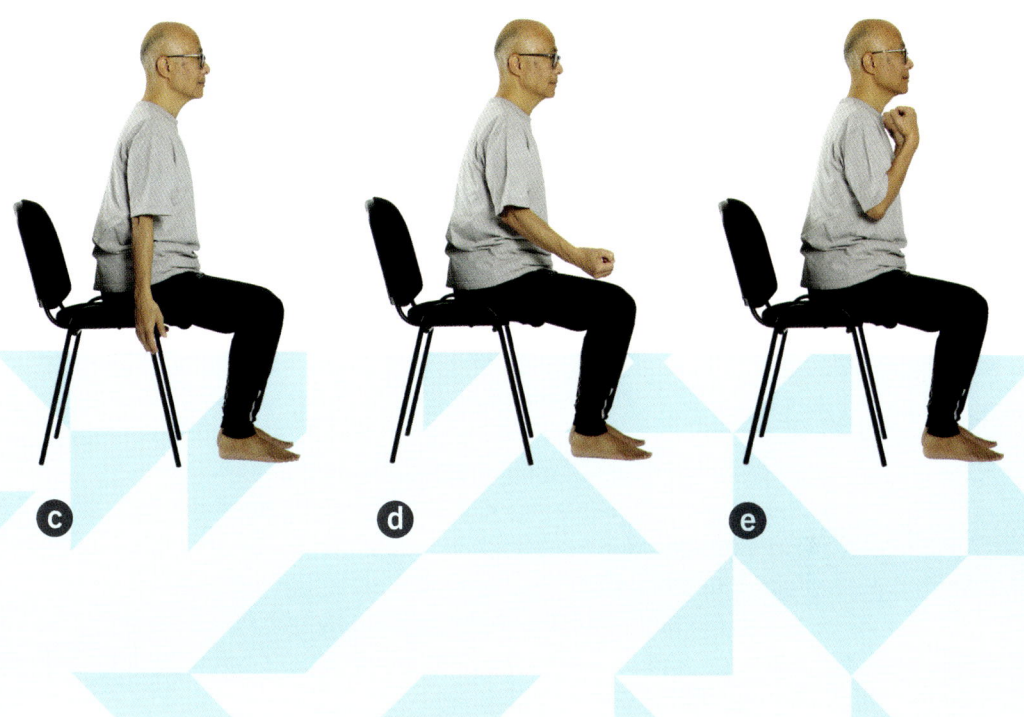

- Now take your arms down to either side of your chair. **c**
- With your fists clenched, breathe in and bending at the elbow lift your arms all the way up to your shoulders, still keeping your elbows close to your ribcage. **d** **e**
- Breathe out and lower them down to the sides of your chair.
- Repeat 8 times.

Shoulder stabilisation means keeping the shoulder steady so that you can move your arm into different positions, as an unstable shoulder can provoke injury – the shoulder being the most flexible joint in the body.

DUMB WAITER (B)

Benefits

This exercise is excellent for relieving any tightness in your chest muscles, and it also mobilises the upper arm and shoulder (the rotator cuff muscles). It is particularly good for shoulder stabilisation and posture. The rotator cuff muscles are a group of muscles in your shoulder that allow for a wide range of movement. If you suffer from a frozen shoulder or arthritis in this area, you might find that this exercise is recommended by your health professional. You'll find the same exercise with a resistance band on page 143 .

Method

- Sit up tall on your chair and engage your abdominal muscles.
- Bend your arms so that your elbows hug your ribcage and your forearms are out in front of you at right angles with your palms facing upwards. **a**
- Breathe in and when you breathe out slowly take your forearms out to the side of your body, keeping your elbows hugging your ribcage. **b**
- Breathe in again and as you breathe out, return your arms gently back to centre.
- Repeat 8 times.

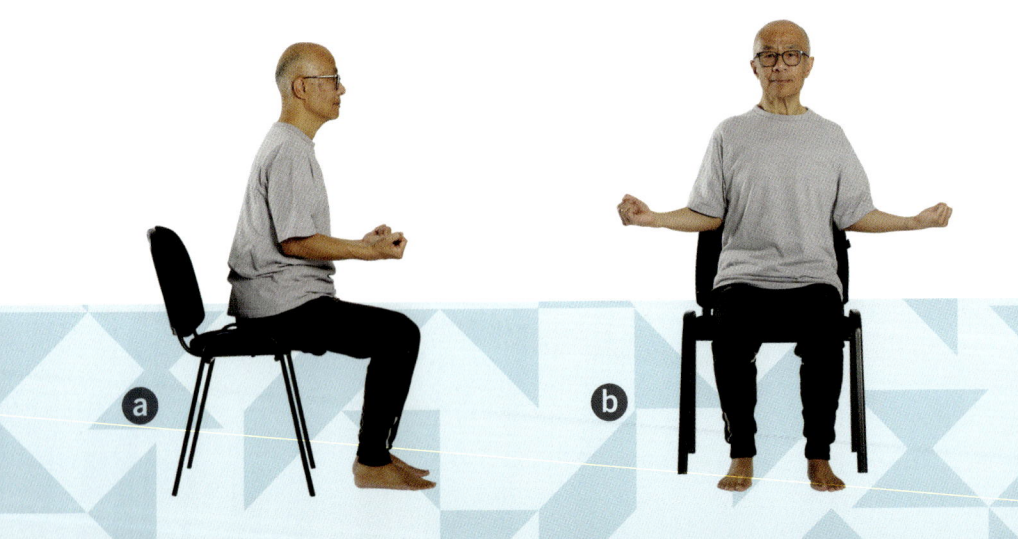

TRICEPS (B)

The triceps muscles sit on the underside of your arms and are often referred to, rather unkindly, as bat or bingo wings. These muscles play an important role in moving your arm away from your body, moving your arms back behind your body and carrying things overhead.

Benefits

Like the biceps, these muscles are important to keep strong and functioning well so that we can go about our everyday activities. If you choose to use hand weights (or tins or water bottles), then have them ready.

Method

- Sit up tall on your chair.
- Take your arms down to either side of your chair, with the back of your arm facing backwards, the front of your arm facing forwards. **a**
- Breathe normally for this exercise.
- Pulse your arms backwards — make quick, small, rhythmic movements back and forth — 16 times. **b**
- Rest and repeat.
- Now bend your elbows to a 90-degree angle with your forearms facing upwards. **c**
- Gently clench your fists if you're not holding weights.
- Perform the same small pulsing movement but this time pulling backwards so that your elbows are pointing and then travelling directly backwards, as if you're elbowing somebody out of the way or pulling something towards you. **d**
- Repeat 16 times.

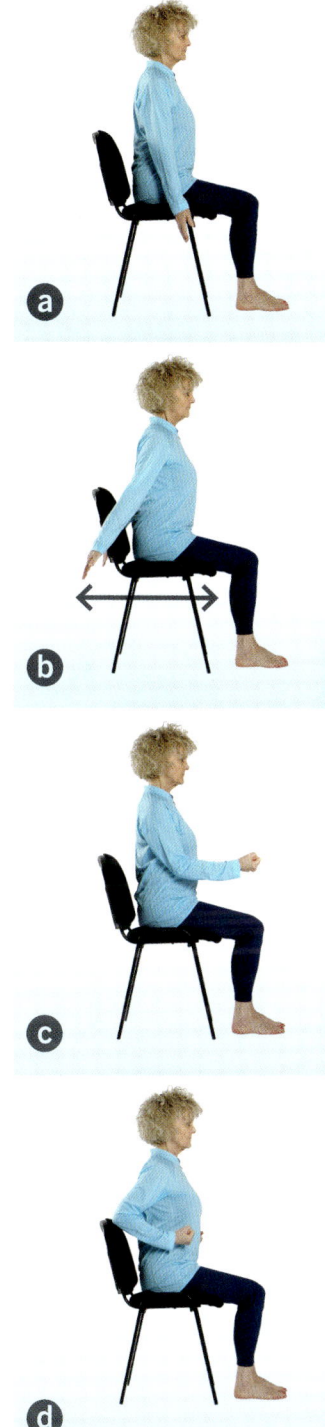

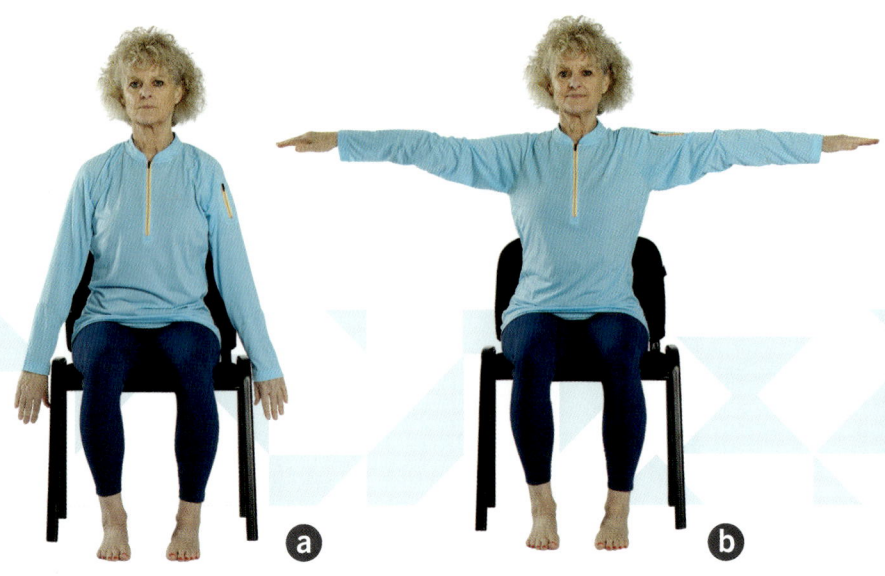

DELTOIDS (B)

These muscles, which sit on the outside of your upper arm, connect the upper arm to your body.

Benefits

They help move your arm in all directions and protect and stabilise your shoulder joint. This exercise will also improve your coordination. If you wish to use hand weights, have them ready.

Method

- Sit up tall on your chair with your arms down by either side. **a**
- Breathe in and as you breathe out raise your arms out to the sides of your body, level with your shoulders like aeroplane wings. **b**
- Hold for a beat.
- Breathe in again and as you breathe out lower them back to the start position.
- Repeat 8 times.

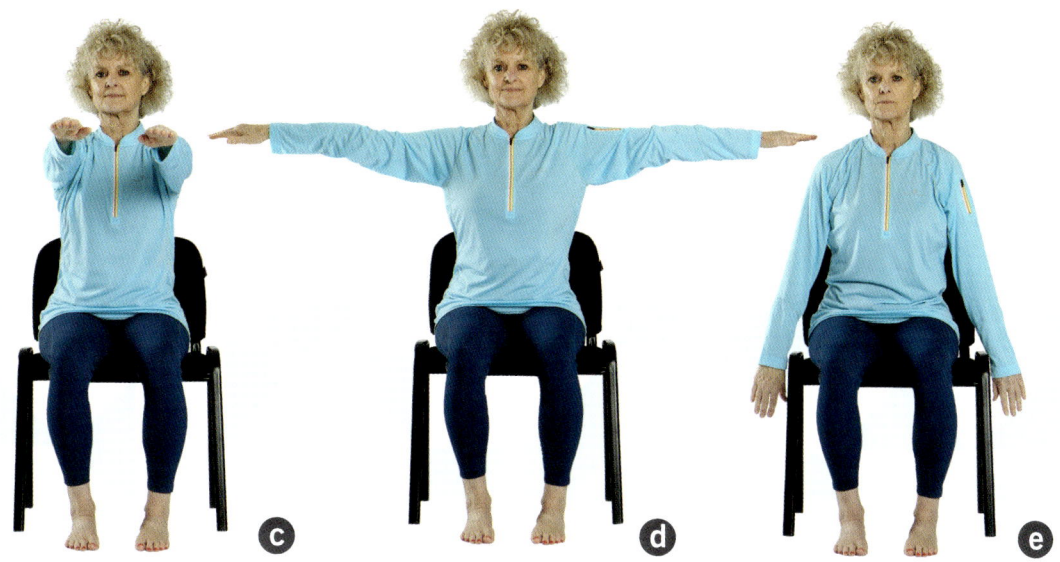

- Rest your arms if they're feeling tired.
- When you're ready, breathe in once again and as you breathe out lift your arms back up into aeroplane wings.
- Breathe in and as you breathe out extend your arms to the front of your body. **c**
- Hold for a beat.
- Breathe in again and as you breathe out return your arms out to the side into aeroplane wings. **d**
- Lower them back down to your sides.
- Let the movement flow: lift to the side, move to the front, hold, return to the side and lower. **e**
- Aim for 8 repetitions, but if your arms tire then rest and pick up again when you're ready.

Note: A journal article in *Age and Ageing* published by Oxford University Press looked at a study of 49 people between the ages of 64 and 91 over a seven-month period where they participated in seated exercise twice weekly. It was noted that after this period of time, there was a noticeable improvement in the participants' ability to stand from sitting, and their grip strength, spinal flexion and general daily living function all benefited from the seated exercise routine.

CACTUS ARMS (B)

Benefits

As well as strengthening the arms and improving the shoulder's range of motion, this exercise opens the chest, rib cage and upper back, helping to strengthen these areas of your body, which will improve your posture. It can also go some way to relieve stiffness in these areas. Use light hand weights (or tins or small bottles of water), if you wish.

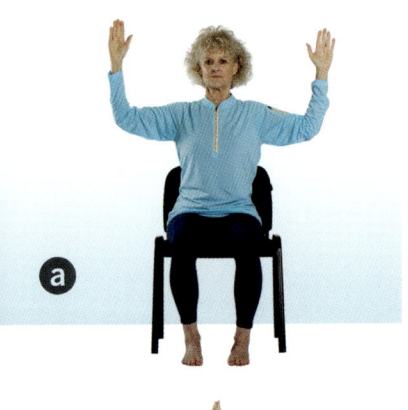

Method

- Sit up tall on your chair.
- Raise your arms to the side of your body, level with your shoulders, and bend at the elbow to form an L-shape, forearms facing upwards, like a cactus, and fingers facing up (unless you're holding weights). **a**
- Take a breath in and as you breathe out, bring your arms in front of your body so that your forearms and the palms of your hands meet in front of your chest. Try not to drop your elbows. **b**
- Hold the posture as you breathe in and then breathe out and return your arms to the side of the body into the L-shape again.
- Repeat 8 times.

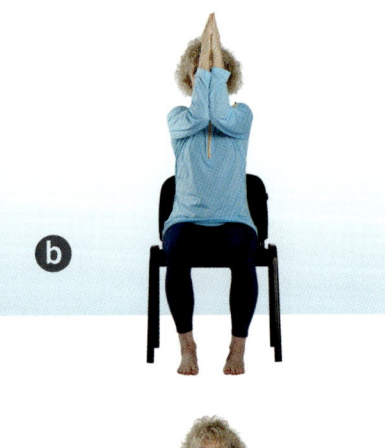

- Rest your arms for a moment and then return them to the cactus position. **a**
- This time drop your forearms downwards, rotating your shoulders as you do so. You might not be able to go far and that's fine. **c**
- Take a breath in again and as you breathe out, lift the forearms up into the cactus position again.
- Repeat 4 times.

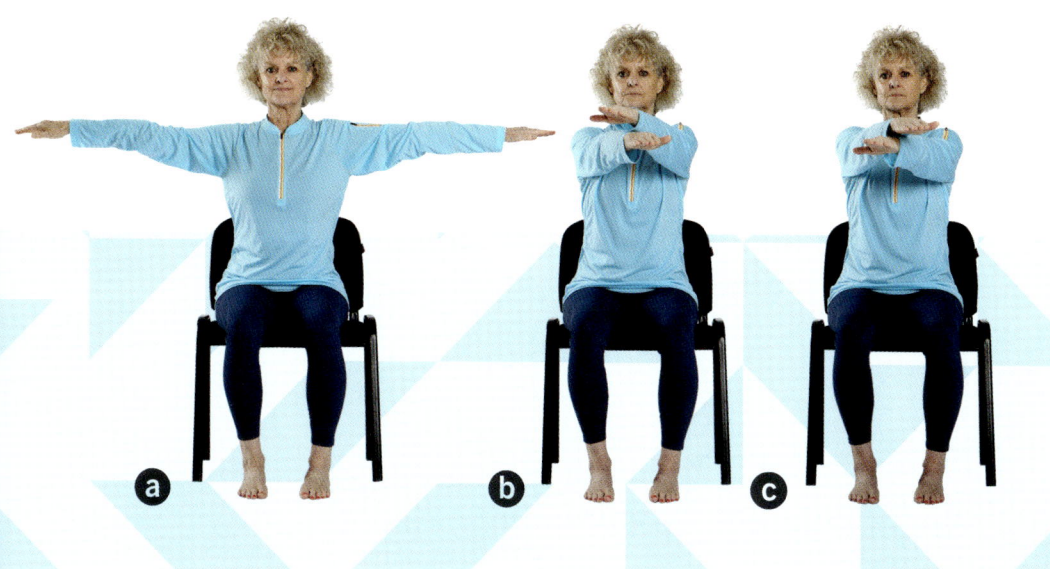

SCISSOR ARMS (B)

Benefits

This exercise will strengthen your chest and upper back, provide shoulder mobility and flexibility and strengthen your arms. If you wish to use light hand weights, then do so.

Method

- Sit up tall on your chair and breathe normally.
- Extend your arms out to the side of your body in the aeroplane wings position. **a**
- Bring your extended arms in front of your torso and criss-cross your wrists 8 times back and forth dynamically. **b** **c**
- Return your arms to aeroplane wings and then take them down to the sides of your chair.
- Repeat 4 times.

SHOULDER AND ARM ROTATIONS (1)

Benefits

This exercise will strengthen your shoulders and arms and improve your coordination. If your arms tire easily, you may want to take a breather halfway through, in which case, do. Hand weights (or small water bottles or tins) will add a more challenging element to the movement.

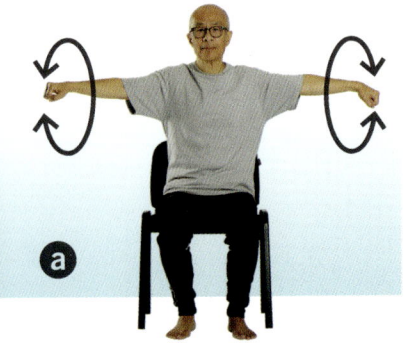

Method

- Sit up tall on your chair.
- Take your arms out to the side of your body in the aeroplane wings position (*see* p. 74).
- Keeping your arms extended to the side, gently rotate your arms from your shoulders, 8 times forwards and 8 times backwards; try not to let them drop lower than your shoulders. **a**

- After you've completed the circling repetitions, bend your elbows and position your arms into the cactus position (*see* p. 76), elbows level with your shoulders and with your fists clenched. **b**
- Take a breath in and as you breathe out, lengthen your arms, hands and fingers above your head. **c**
- Breathe in again with your arms still extended above your head and as you breathe out, return your arms, with control, to the cactus position, elbows level with your shoulders once more and with your fists clenched.
- Repeat 8 times, increasing the repetitions when you feel ready to do so.

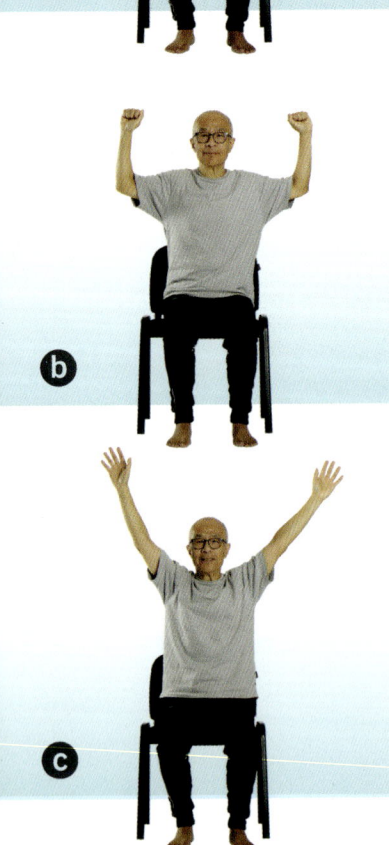

NUMBER 8, GARDEN GATE (I)

Benefits

This exercise will challenge your coordination and improve concentration as well as improve arm and shoulder mobility. Make sure you have space in front of your chair to extend your arms and wave them around.

Do not grow old, no matter how long you live. Never cease to stand like curious children before the Great Mystery into which we were born.'

Albert Einstein

Method

- Sit up tall on your chair.
- Breathe normally for this exercise but be aware that because you are concentrating hard, there is a tendency to hold your breath, so try to incorporate conscious, mindful breathing.
- Extend one arm in front of your body and draw a figure of 8 in the air with it, 4 times, mobilising the whole arm and shoulder as you do so. **a**
- Reverse the movement, so you're going back the other way, 4 times. Reversing the movement can sometimes be more challenging!
- Repeat with the other arm.

- Now take both arms out in front of your torso and move them both together in a figure of 8 for 4 repetitions. **b**
- Reverse the movement, 4 times.

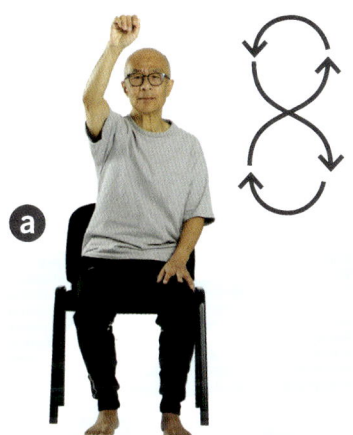

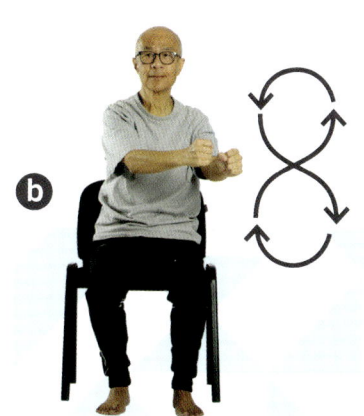

BREASTSTROKE SWIMMING (1)

Benefits

This movement will work your shoulders, triceps (back of your arms) and chest muscles, and it is also a coordination exercise. If you enjoy swimming, then you will recognise this as breaststroke.

Make sure you have space to the side of your chair and there is nothing in the way of your hands or arms in front of your torso.

Method

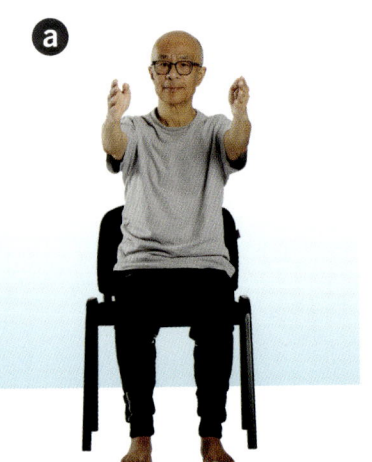

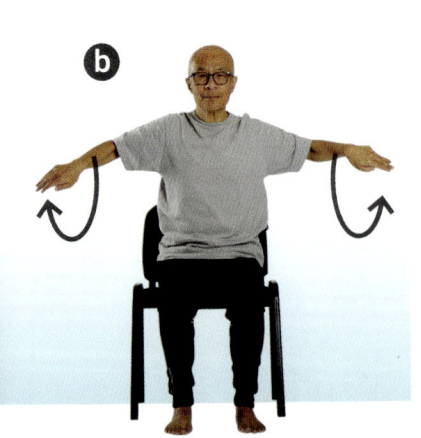

- Sit up tall on your chair.
- Extend both your arms out in front of your torso, palms facing each other. **a**
- Breathe in and as you breathe out, sweep your arms around to the side of your body rotating your arms as you do so (imagine the water being pushed back by the palms of your hands). **b**
- Bend your elbows, rotate your arms once again and sweep forwards bringing the palms of your hands together and back to the start position.
- Take another breath in here and breathe out as you once again perform the breaststroke action.
- Perform 8 repetitions slowly.
- If you find it hard to coordinate the breathing with this exercise, then just breathe normally; make sure you don't hold your breath.

CRAWL SWIMMING (B)

Benefits

This movement will work your shoulders, triceps (back of your arms), biceps and chest muscles, and it is also a coordination exercise. If you have shoulder problems, take it easy and make the movement small. If you enjoy swimming, then you will recognise this as the crawl.

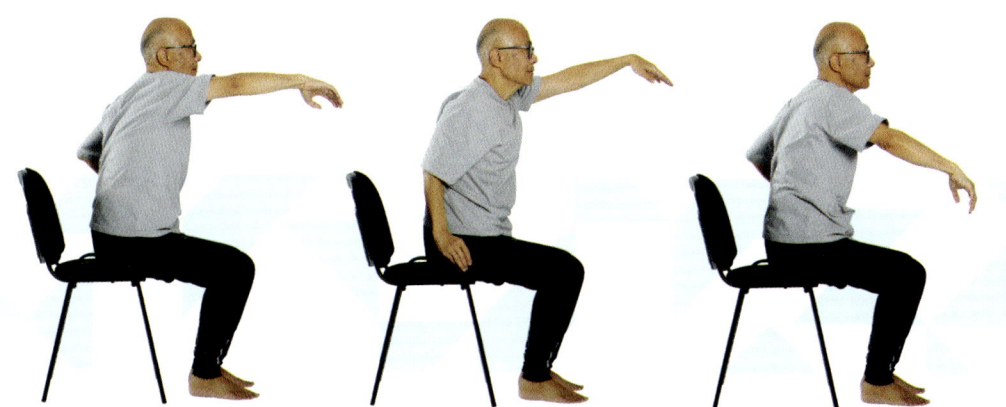

Method

- Sit up tall on your chair.
- Breathe normally for this exercise. You'll perform it dynamically as you would in a swimming pool.
- Lift up your right arm and make a 'crawl' stroke across your body, keeping your fingers relaxed.
- Repeat on the left.
- Alternate the arms, maybe visualising yourself swimming towards a lovely beach!
- Perform 16 times in total — 8 on each arm — and then rest your arms, rotating your shoulders if you need to.

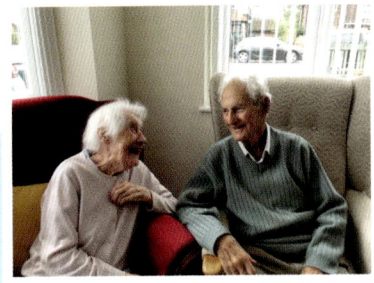

CASE STUDY

Audrey and Wreford Gibbs
BOTH AGED 92

Audrey: 'I find Chair Pilates and Yoga quite useful, especially for my shoulders that are stiff – I sometimes do the arm and shoulder exercises at home but then forget! I have an arthritic knee, so it's really good to keep it moving so it doesn't stiffen up and get too painful. But I enjoy the chair exercises.'

Wreford: 'The exercises are enjoyable and the sit-to-stand exercise [see p. 128] is particularly useful to do – it takes me a while, but once I've done a couple, the body seems to know what to do. I do keep mobile by working in the garden quite a bit, but this sort of exercise is something we've both got to keep at; it should be a continuous thing, daily. You can always find a few minutes somewhere in your day to do it. But having said that, basically, we are both bone idle!'

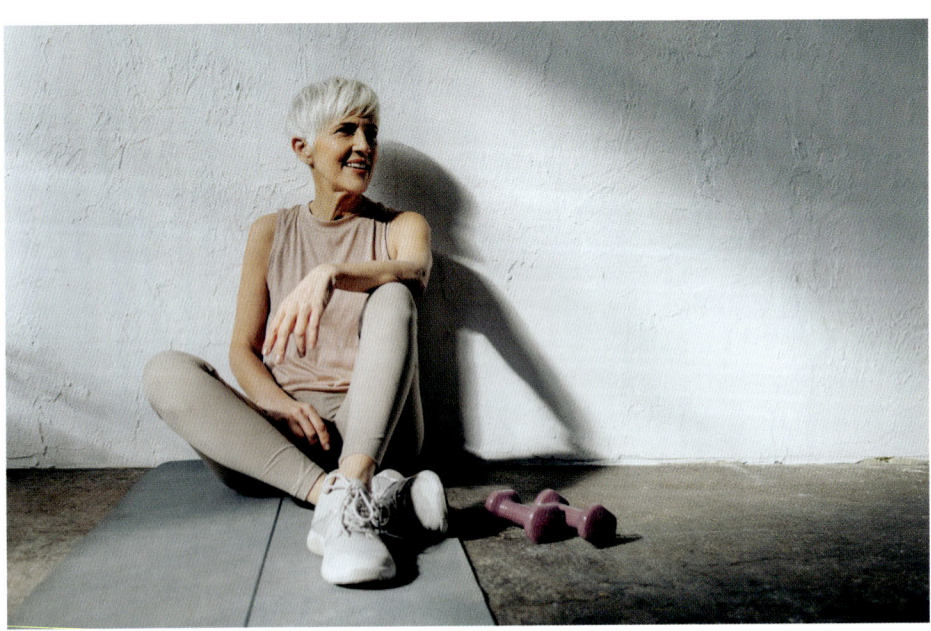

ROW, ROW, ROW (I)

Benefits

This movement will strengthen your upper back, arms and shoulders; and if you've ever rowed a boat, this is exactly what you will be doing here. An added bonus of this exercise is that you will also be working your abdominal muscles as you move your torso back and forth.

Method

- Sit up tall on your chair and move yourself a little further forwards on the seat.
- Extend your arms in front of your torso and lean slightly forwards on your chair, bringing the arms close together.
- Breathe in and as you breathe out, imagine grabbing an oar in each hand. **a**
- Pull backwards, bending your elbows and squeezing your shoulder blades together as you pull your imaginary oars through the water. **b**
- Begin to sit up straighter before leaning back a little as you 'pull'.
- Shift forwards on your chair once again and repeat the rowing movement 8 times.

If you find the coordination of this exercise challenging, then just imagine you are sitting in a rowing boat, oars in hand, rowing towards shore, and try not to overthink it!

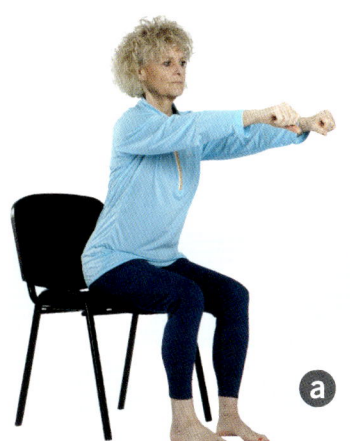

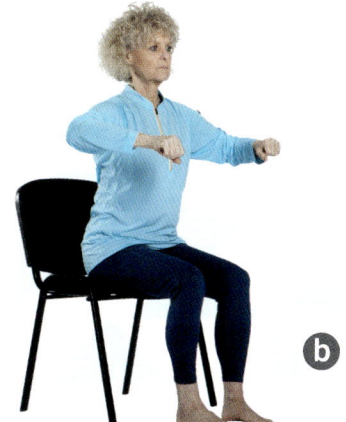

PACK A PUNCH 1 (B)

Benefits

This exercise will work your arms and back muscles and over time increase flexibility. It can be performed dynamically, or in slow motion to make more of the lengthening motion with your arms. It's up to you.

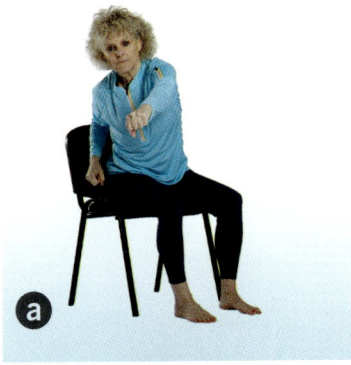

Method

- Sit up tall on your chair.
- Lightly clench your fist (or hold a small hand weight, or water bottle or tin, if you wish).
- If you choose to perform this exercise slowly, and I would suggest you do if you're new to this, breathe normally and make a slow-motion punching movement: extend your arm across your body, gently twisting your torso. **a**
- Return your arm to the start position.
- Repeat on the other side.
- Continue, alternating the arms and punching out either side of your body in slow motion. Don't forget to keep breathing. **b** **c**
- Repeat 16 times.

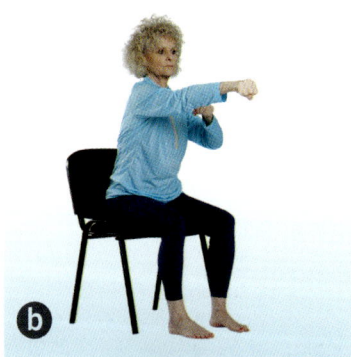

If you find the slow-motion version challenging, then go at a speed that works for you.

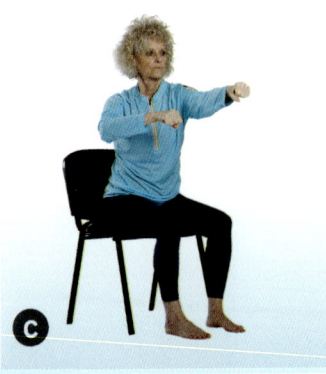

PACK A PUNCH 2 (I)

Benefits

This is more of a power move than Pack a Punch 1, as you'll be punching above your head and using more arm, chest and back muscle force. If you choose to use small hand weights (or small water bottles or tins) please take good care and make sure that you grip them well when they are above your head!

Method

- Sit up tall on your chair.
- Take your arms down to the side of your chair and lightly clench your fists.
- Breathe in and as you breathe out raise one arm and punch the air above your head. **a**
- Breathe in and return your arm to the start position as you breathe out. Repeat on the other side. **b**
- Continue to alternate the arms punching the air slowly, or if you prefer, make the repetitions faster.
- If you do make the repetitions faster, then you'll need to breathe normally.

- If you wish to make the exercise even more challenging, lift the opposite leg at the same time. This adds an element of coordination to the exercise – opposite arm to leg. **c**
- Repeat 16 times.

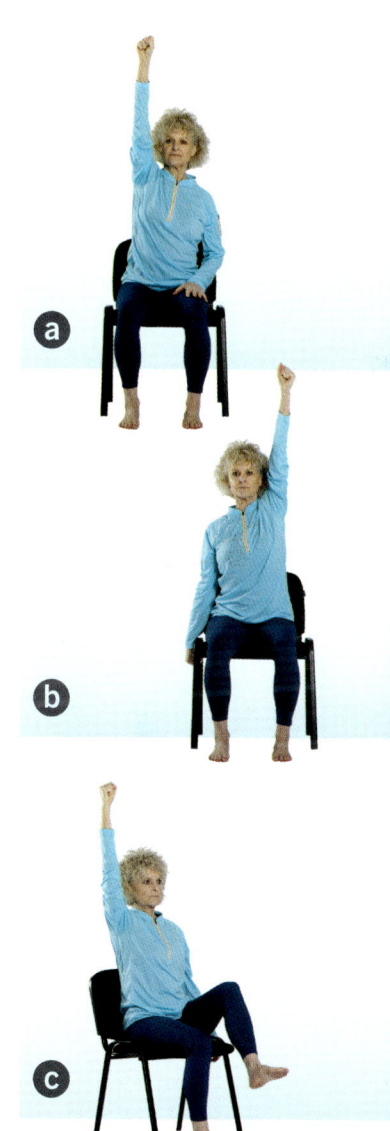

CHAPTER 11

ABDOMINAL MUSCLES

It may surprise you to know that you can exercise your abdominal muscles while sitting in a chair, but you can! What's important is that you engage your abdominal muscles as you perform the movement. If you need reminding about how to do this effectively, then turn to page 24.

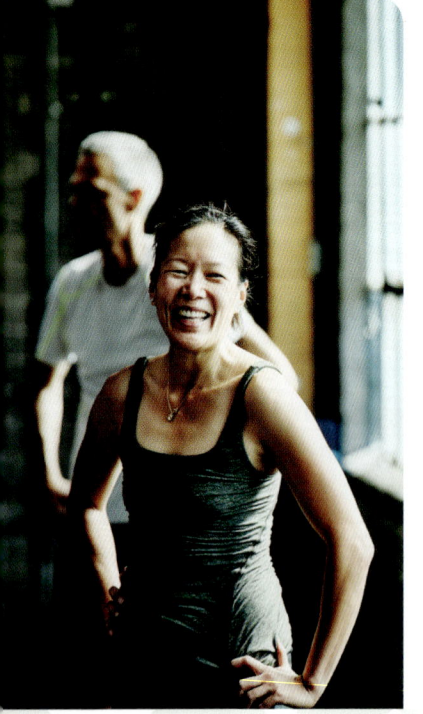

Benefits

These exercises will not only strengthen those tummy muscles, but also, over time, tone them and improve your posture; and if you suffer lower back ache, they may help relieve this problem as your abdominal muscles begin to strengthen. See page 24 for more information about how important your abdominal muscles are, specifically your transversus abdominus, in relation to your back.

PULL THOSE ABS IN (B)

Benefits

This is a simple and effective exercise for your abdominal muscles. Not only can you perform it while seated, but also you can perform this exercise in the supermarket queue, standing waiting for a bus or when doing the washing up, and nobody will know you're doing it.

Method

- Sit up tall on your chair, lengthen through the spine with your feet on the floor below your knees.
- Place your hands on your thighs. Find your neutral spine (*see* p. 23).
- All you are going to do is pull your abdominal muscles in: not to the third notch on your belt (*see* p. 25) but to the tenth notch.
- Breathe in and as you breathe out pull those tummy muscles in as tight as you can.
- Hold as you breathe in again and then release on the exhale. Nothing else should move; your spine should remain lengthened and strong.
- Repeat 4 times or more, depending on how you feel.
- Hold for longer if you feel able.

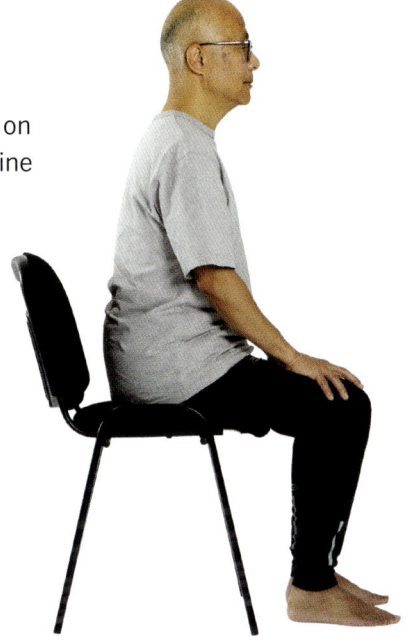

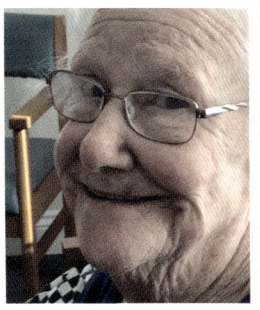

CASE STUDY

BETTE KURKA
AGE 94

'Chair exercise is good for you; I love it. I've got lazy and forgotten where my tummy muscles are! So it's good to be made to do them – I like the chest stretch too; it feels like I need it, as I tend to sit a lot these days.'

STIR THE CAULDRON (B)

Benefits

This exercise will work the middle of your torso — all your abdominal muscles including your obliques (your waist). It's also a mobility exercise for your spine.

Method

- Sit up tall on your chair and engage your abdominal muscles.
- Extend both of your arms out in front of you — imagine that you are grabbing on to a large stick or ladle that is going to stir a big cauldron of soup. **a**
- Take a breath in and as you breathe out start to stir your large pot with your imaginary stick, circling your torso round and round with your arms increasing the circle with each rotation. Keep your bottom glued to your seat and your feet firmly on the floor. **b** **c**
- As your rotations or stirring motions increase in size, you'll find that your torso will go backwards and forwards and from side to side.
- Rotate 4 times to the right and then 4 times to the left.

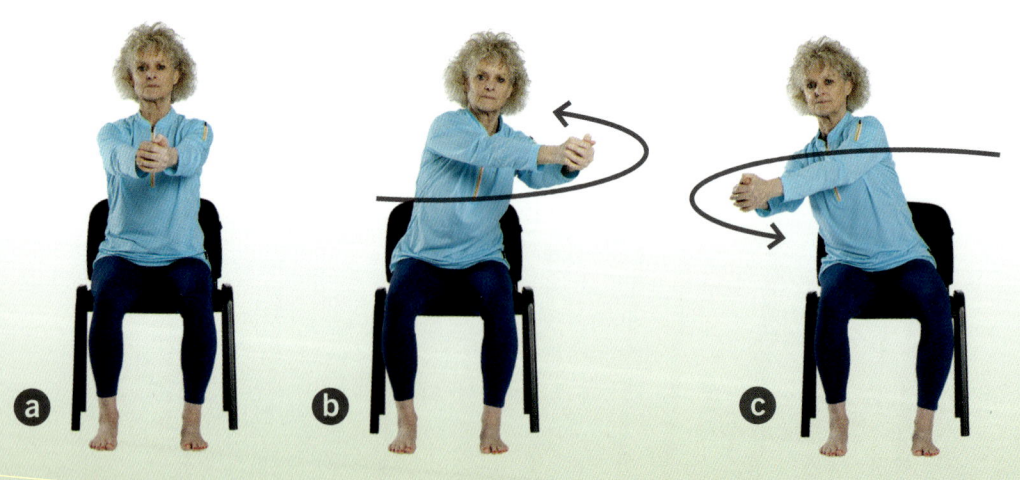

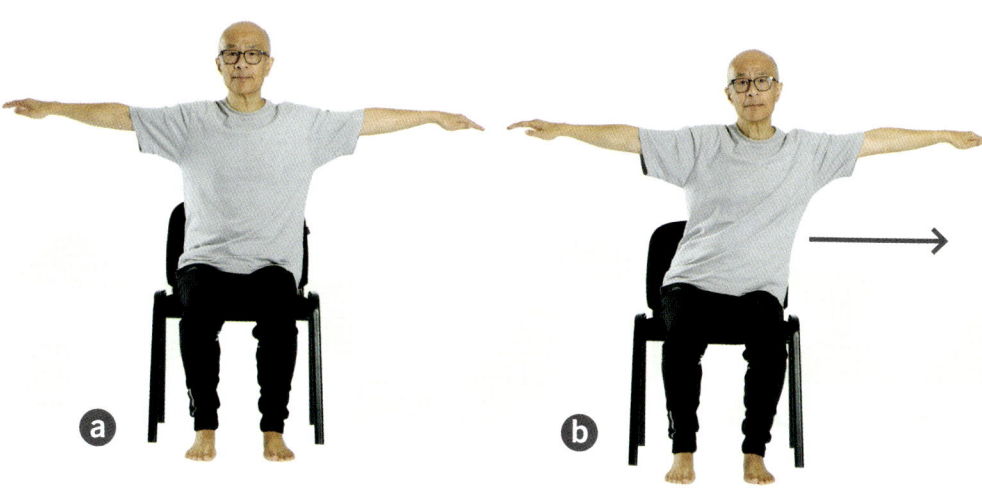

OBLIQUES (B)

Your obliques — waist muscles — help you to bend and twist and are important in protecting your spine, like the other abdominal muscles.

Benefits

By strengthening your oblique muscles, you will improve your posture. If your balance isn't particularly good, one reason for this can be that these muscles, which are part of your core muscles, are weak. Strengthening these muscles can go some way to improving your balance.

Method

- Sit up tall on your chair and engage your abdominal muscles.
- Extend your arms to the side of your body like aeroplane wings. **a**
- Take a breath in and as you breathe out, and moving from your waist, reach your right arm and fingertips towards the left side of the room as if you are trying to touch the wall on the other side. **b**
- Breathe in as you hold this lengthening position.
- Breathe out and return to sitting upright.
- Repeat on the other side.
- Repeat 8 times.

SIT-UP AND CRUNCH TIME (1)

This exercise is a seated adaptation of the stomach crunch or sit-up that is most often performed while lying on your back.

Benefits

By performing this exercise you'll be strengthening and toning your tummy muscles.

Method

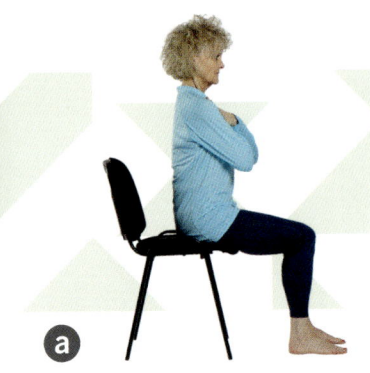

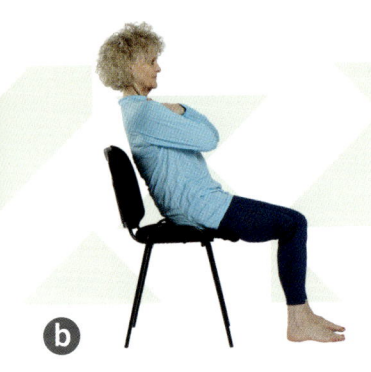

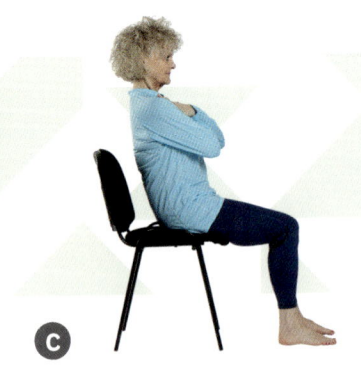

- Shift yourself to the edge of your chair with your feet and knees slightly further forwards.
- Cross your arms across your chest.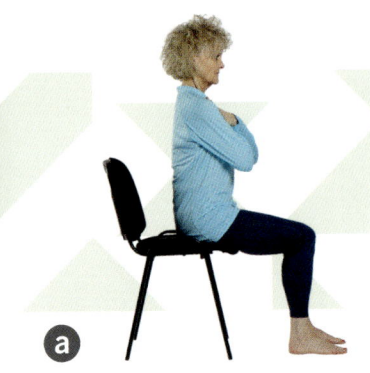
- Lean yourself back so that you are sitting at an angle, but keep your back straight.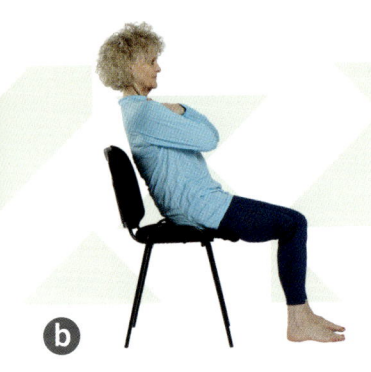
- Engage your abdominal muscles and/or your pelvic floor muscles and try to keep your shoulders relaxed.
- Breathe in and as you breathe out, lift your torso from the leaning back position to an upright position, all the while keeping your back straight.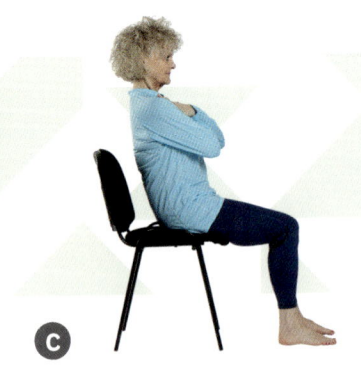
- Breathe in and as you breathe out, slowly and with control, lean yourself gently back again, keeping your spine straight.
- Lean back to the point where you feel your tummy muscles working. You'll know when that is.
- Breathe in and as you breathe out lift yourself back up to the upright position once again — keep those abdominal muscles pulled in and your back straight.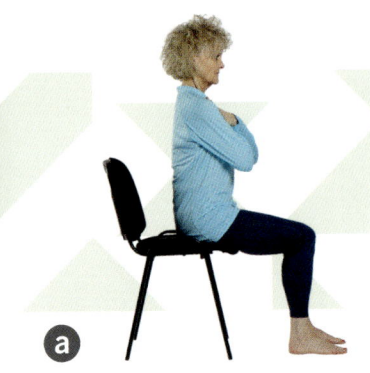

- If you want to feel your abdominal muscles working, you can place one hand on your stomach while you do this exercise — you should feel the muscles engage under the palm of your hand, which is proof if you need it!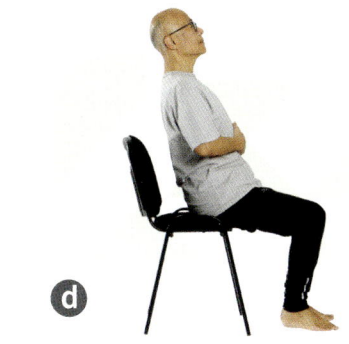
- Repeat 8 times.

CRUNCH TIME 2 (1)

Method

- Sit up tall towards the edge of your chair.
- Place your hands on either side of the chair.
- Breathe normally for this exercise as you'll be performing it dynamically. But do remember to breathe and not hold your breath!
- Lift your right knee up and towards your chest, leaning slightly into it as you do so.
- Return your leg and foot to the ground.
- Repeat on the other side.
- Repeat 8 times.

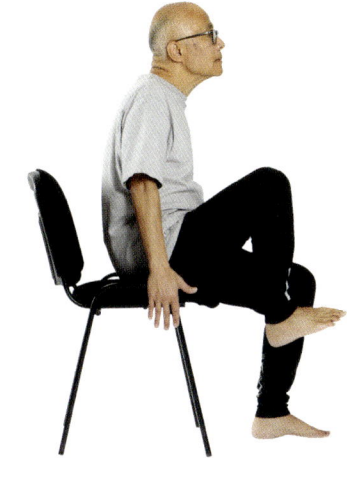

Variations

- If you'd like to make the exercise a little more challenging, then lift both knees up together — you'll find that you naturally lean back as you raise your knees and you will need to keep the palms of your hands glued to the sides of your chair for stability.
- Repeat 8 times.

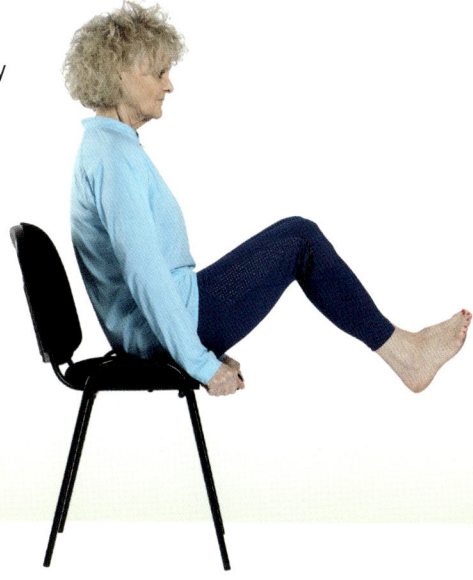

LOWER ABDOMINAL MUSCLES (I)

Method

- Sit up tall on your chair, and lengthen through the spine but with your feet slightly wider than hip-width apart.
- Clasp your hands together, making a fist, and extend your arms in front of you. **a**
- Take your hands down to the inside of your right knee and press against it, allow your knee to press back into your fist in response. **b**
- Hold for the silent count of four, breathing normally, and release.
- Repeat on the other side. As you perform this exercise you should feel your lower abdominal muscles contract.
- Repeat 4 times.

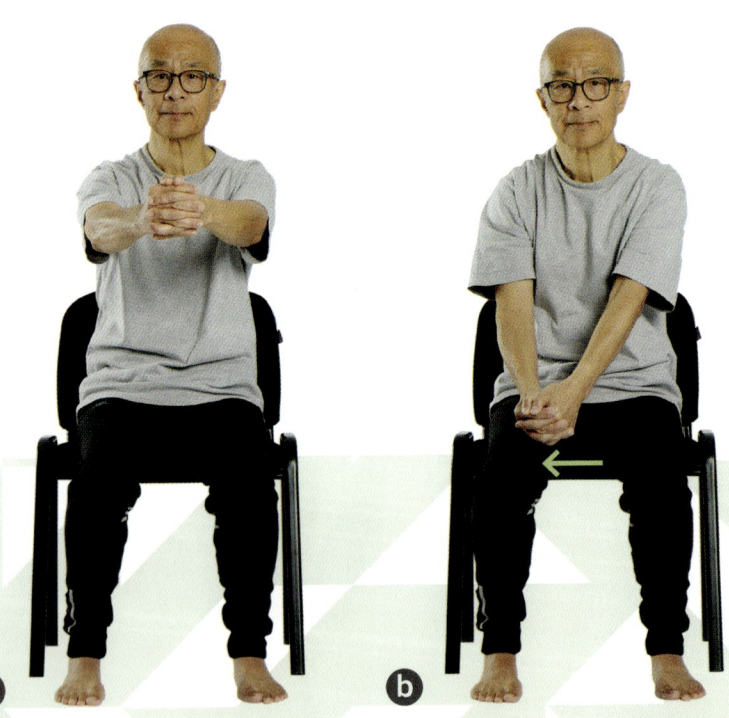

CHAPTER 12

GLUTES

It might surprise you to know that, like the abdominal muscles, your glutes (your bottom muscles) can be worked while sitting down.

Benefits

We need our bottom muscles to remain strong to keep us moving easily and to help us to remain upright. These muscles also support the lower back, particularly when lifting something, and by keeping them strong we can also go some way to preventing knee injuries.

BUTT CLENCH 1 (B)

Yes, really, that is all you need to do — clench your buttocks.

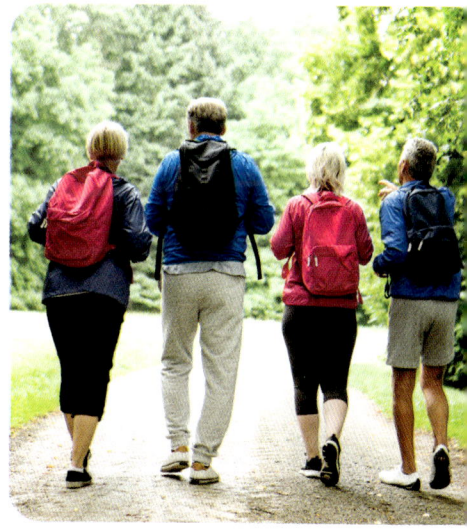

Method

- Sit up tall on your chair with a neutral spine (*see* p. 23) with your feet parallel and on the floor below your knees.
- For this exercise breathe normally, but be aware of any tension in your body, particularly your jaw, which might want to clench at the same time as your buttocks!
- Engage your abdominal muscles and/or pelvic floor muscles.

You can't help getting older, but you don't have to get old.'

George Burns

- Place your hands on your thighs and keep your shoulders relaxed.
- Simply, clench your bottom muscles together. You'll feel yourself rise up off the chair a little each time you do it and it might feel odd to begin with, but it really works!
- Clench your bottom muscles quickly 8 times, rest and then repeat.

BUTT CLENCH 2 (I)

This exercise will challenge those important bottom muscles further. Make sure before you attempt this that you've mastered Butt Clench 1 described above.

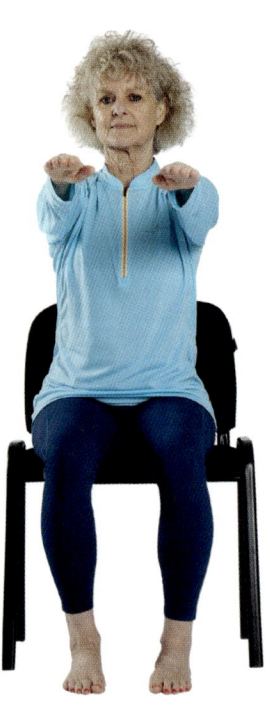

Benefits

If you sit for long periods of time, then your buttock muscles will weaken and forget how to work. Another reason we can become more prone to falls as we age is weak gluteals, but they help us to stand, walk and balance, and strong buttock muscles can improve posture. So don't forget to include them in your exercise routine, however ridiculous this may feel!

Method

- Sit up tall on your chair, lengthen through the spine with your feet shoulder-width apart.
- Breathe normally for this exercise but make sure you don't hold your breath, grit your teeth or clench your jaw as you engage your butt!
- Extend your arms out in front of your torso.
- Clench your buttocks and hold for a silent count of four and then release.
- Repeat 4 times.

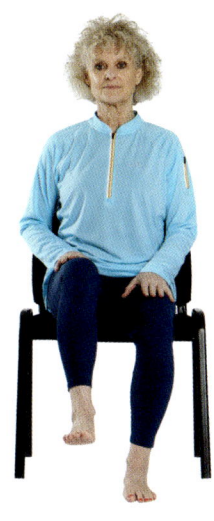

- Taking this exercise one step further, try clenching your buttock muscles and lifting one foot slightly off the floor at the same time.
- Try engaging your abdominal muscles and/or pelvic floor muscles at the same time. You might in fact feel them engage automatically as you work your buttock muscles.

You'll find another glute exercise among the standing exercises using the chair as a prop on page 139.

CASE STUDY

JENNIFER COCKS
AGE 78

'I have been doing Chair Pilates and Yoga with Harri for some time. I used to do floor Pilates before lockdown but moved, so now I stick to online video classes. I started with the Chair Pilates and Yoga as I was struggling with problems in my right knee. At that stage it really helped, improving mobility in my knee. But my knee was getting progressively worse; I only had moderate to severe arthritis, so this did not qualify me for an operation. A while later the knee began curling in towards my left leg, and I was heavily knock-kneed. After a series of X-rays I was recommended a total knee replacement; the left-hand side of my knee was OK, but the right-hand side was 'bone-on-bone'. I continued with chair exercises until the operation and did my physiotherapist's exercises every day as well. Once I had the operation I was out of bed and on crutches next morning. It was important to me to continue the Chair Pilates and Yoga sessions with Harri, as I found that the knee and leg exercises helped my mobility. My physio recommended that I should do the exercises he had prescribed for the first three weeks but then agreed that I could restart Harri's classes and also continue with his harder exercises; I found that when doing both sets of exercises, I was regaining mobility really quickly. By the sixth week after my operation, I was off sticks completely and walking almost normally.'

CHAPTER 13

LEGS, KNEES AND HIPS

Being inactive causes our bones and muscles to lose strength and flexibility — there's more information about what happens to us as we age and on losing muscle mass on page 12. General wear and tear can occur, too, particularly in the knees and hips. Osteoarthritis and other joint conditions can be debilitating, painful and, for so many, the reason inactivity sets in. But by keeping the muscles around the hips, knees and ankles strong with the simple, low-impact seated exercises in this chapter, you'll find that any stiffness and pain will reduce as you gently increase the joint's range of movement and strengthen the surrounding muscles.

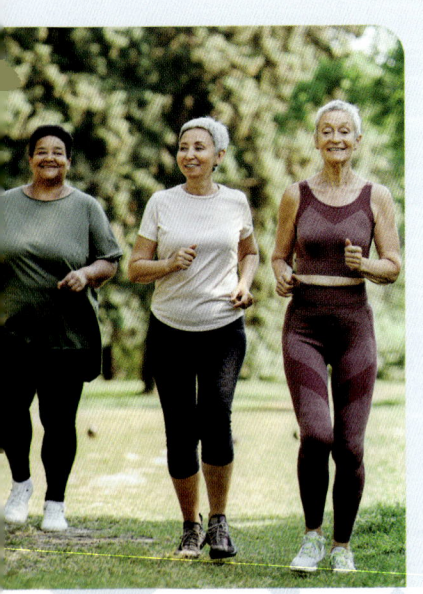

HEEL SLIDES (B)

Benefits

This simple exercise is good for knee mobility, especially if you're recovering from an injury or operation on your knee (once given the go-ahead by your health professional — see page 40 for physiotherapist advice). Traditionally this would be performed lying down on the floor, but it is just as effective sitting on a chair. Bare feet are best: if you wear shoes, the slide won't be as even. This will also depend on your floor — the slide of your heel may be smooth (laminate, tiles, lino) or require more effort (carpet).

Method

- Sit up tall on your chair and rest your hands on your thighs.
- Flex your right foot, so that your toes are pointing upwards and your heel is the only part of your foot on the ground. **a**
- Take a breath in and as you breathe out gently slide your heel forwards and directly in front of you as far as it will go, mobilising your knee. **b**
- Breathe in and as you breathe out gently ease the leg back to the start position.
- Repeat 8 times on both sides.
- If you have a laminate or wooden floor, you can place a duster or tea towel under your heel to make the sliding back and forth smoother. **c**

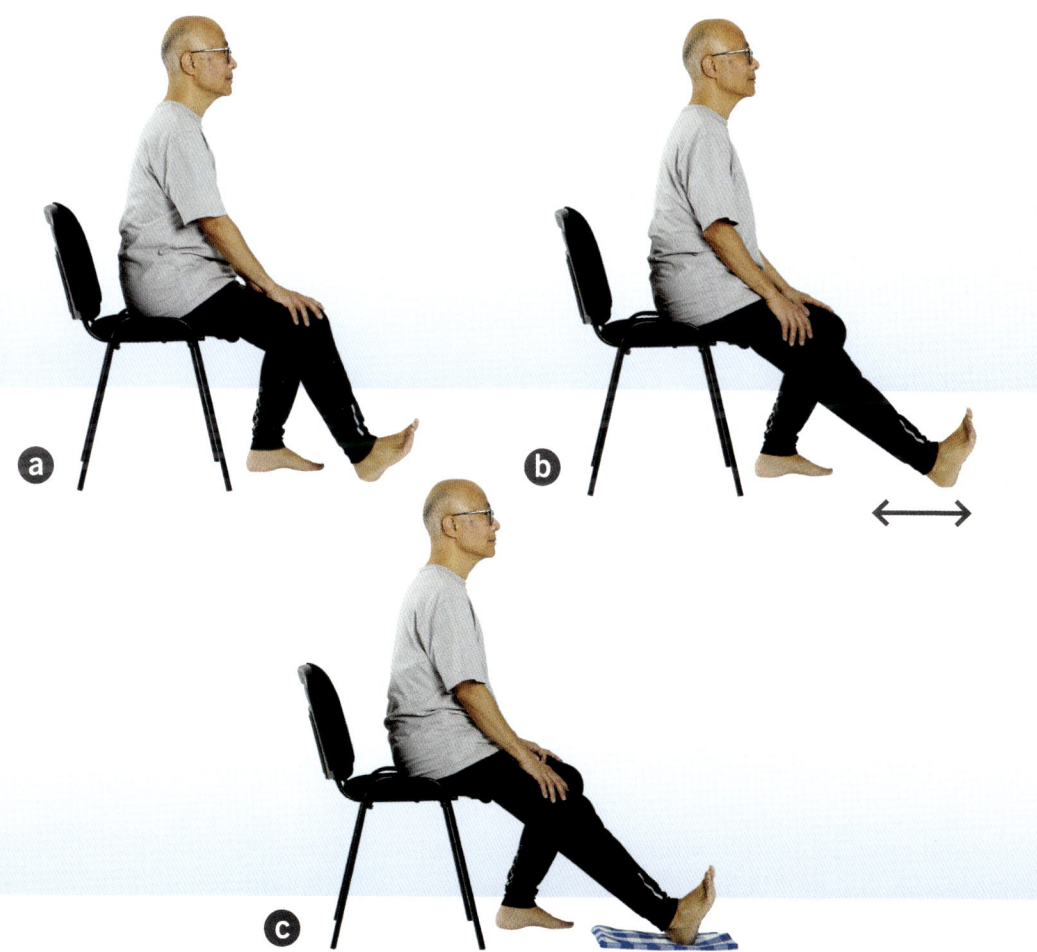

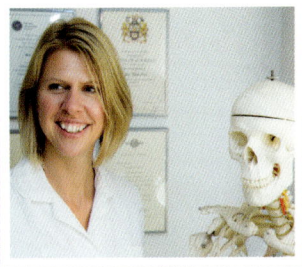

PROFESSIONAL ADVICE

OSTEOPATH, JANE KAUSHAL

Jane says:

'Many injuries to the ankles and knees arise because of poor balance. If you have ever sprained your ankle, the proprioceptors (joint position sensors) in your ankle ligaments will not be as efficient at detecting where your ankle is in space. This means that other structures in the lower extremity take the strain instead, especially when you are walking on uneven ground. Chair-based Pilates and yoga can improve proprioception, which will reduce unnecessary strain on joints and help prevent injury. Your ability to balance decreases naturally with age, so you need to work to maintain or even improve this. Importantly, improved proprioception and balance will help to prevent falls, and balance exercises using the chair as a prop can certainly help in that respect. Falling in later life is bad news for many reasons, so anything we can do to prevent this is very helpful indeed!'

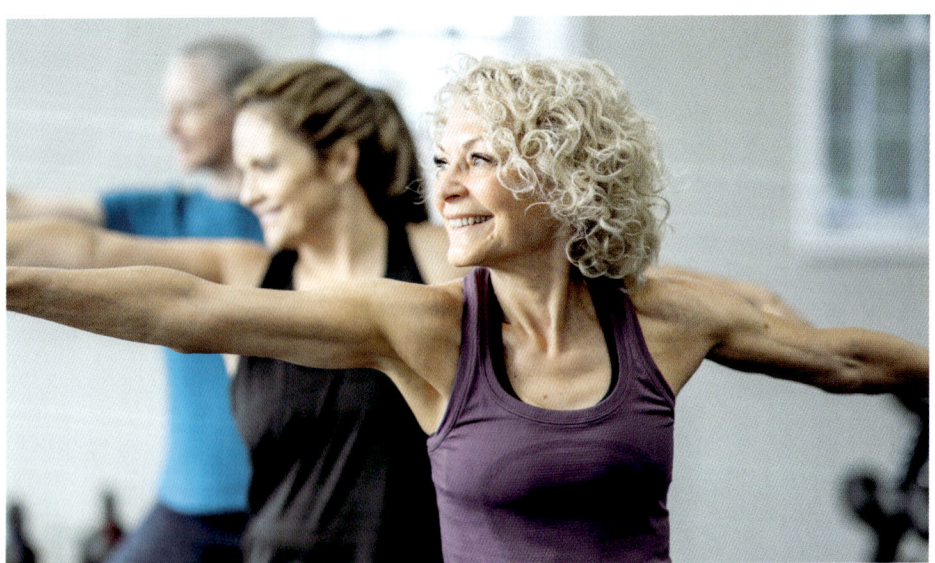

KNEE LIFTS (B)

Traditionally in Pilates, this exercise is performed while standing up and includes balance, but we can perform an adapted version while sitting.

Benefits

This exercise will help strengthen your knees, hips and thighs and strengthen your abdominal muscles. The movement will help with walking as you will mimic the motion despite being seated.

Method

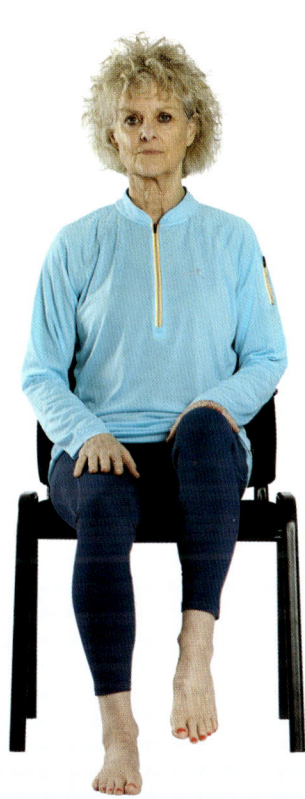

- Sit up tall on your chair.
- Keep your arms and shoulders relaxed with your arms either by your side or your hands resting on your thighs. If you do rest your hands on your thighs, you will be adding just a little extra weight to your leg – which is fine!
- Breathe in and as you breathe out, raise one knee up, keeping it at a 90-degree angle. Imagine a vertical line from your knee to your foot as you lift it up. You may be able to lift the foot only a tiny bit off the floor, which is fine, or you may be able to lift your knee up parallel with your hip or even higher. Just work to a level that feels comfortable for you.
- Try not to collapse in your centre, stay lengthened through the spine throughout and then return your foot to the floor.
- Repeat 8 times with this leg and then move to the other.

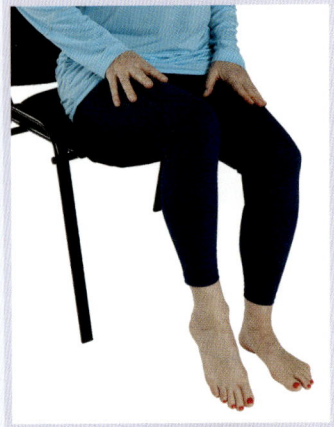

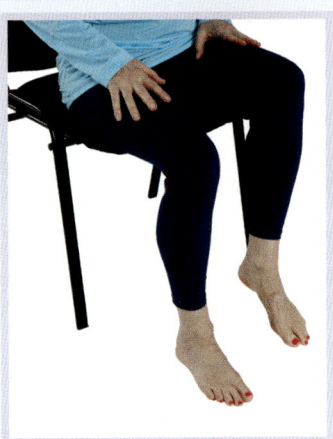

TREACLE FEET (B)

Benefits

A simple exercise to get those legs, knees and hips moving more and to warm them up before attempting the other exercises — imagine you're walking through treacle or mud and the soles of your feet are sticky and therefore difficult to lift up!

Method

- Sit up tall on your chair.
- Relax your shoulders and rest the palms of your hands on your thighs, or place the palms of your hands beside your hips on the chair.
- Breathe normally for this exercise.
- Imagining your feet are heavy and slightly stuck, so it requires more effort, lift one foot up in a walking motion.
- Place it back down on the floor, then lift the other one up.
- Repeat 16 leg lifts in total.

MARCHING ARMS AND LEGS (B)

Benefits

Marching your arms and legs together is not only a coordination exercise, but it will also help you with walking and climbing stairs, as it strengthens your hip flexors (these help raise your legs when you walk) and thighs. This exercise can also be quite energising.

Method

- Sit up tall on your chair, move yourself slightly forwards in your seat.
- Take a breath in and as you breathe out, raise your right knee and your left arm, bending at the elbow to form a walking motion.
- Repeat on the other side — opposite hand to leg.
- Complete 16 repetitions in total.
- If you find the suggested breathing makes the exercise too slow and therefore somewhat challenging, just breathe normally and perform the movement at a speed that suits you.

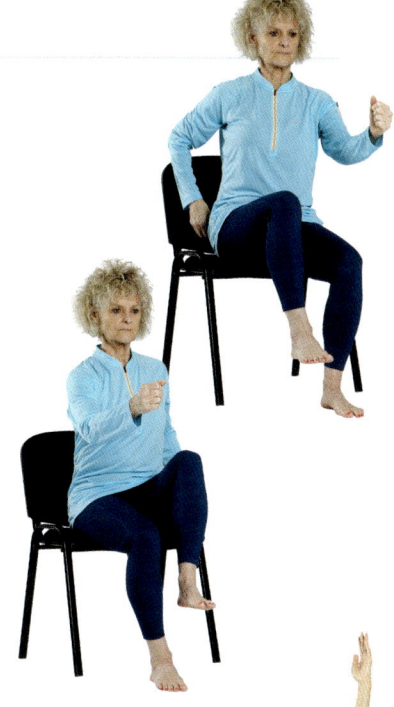

MARCHING ARMS AND LEGS (1)

Method

Once you have repeated the 16 repetitions, progress to raising the arm in the air as the knee is lifted, adding a more demanding movement.

- Take your arms down to the side of your chair.
- Breathe in and as you breathe out, raise your right knee and raise your left arm straight in the air above your head. If you find you're unable to lift your arm very high, then just raise it to wherever it reaches; don't force it — over time and with practice, any mobility issues will improve.
- Breathe in as you hold for a beat.
- Breathe out again and lower the leg and arm back down to the start position.
- Repeat on the other side.
- Repeat 8 times, alternating both arms and legs.
- If you find the breathing makes the movement too slow and awkward, breathe normally and go at your own speed.

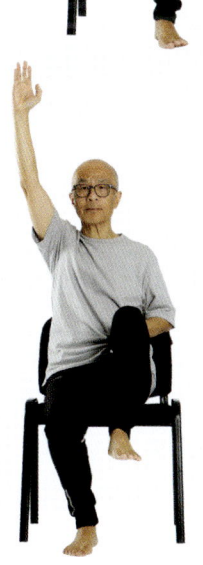

LEG EXTENSIONS (1)

This exercise concentrates on the quads — your thigh muscles.

Benefits

By strengthening your thigh muscles you will be improving the stability of your knee, which in turn can help you be less prone to knee injuries. When your thigh muscles are strong and functioning well, you'll find walking and climbing stairs easier and good posture and balance will be maintained.

Method

- Sit up tall on your chair.
- Breathe normally for this exercise as the movement is quite fast.
- Extend your right leg out in front of you, lifting it off the floor, and flex your foot.
- Keeping your leg straight, gently pulse: small dynamic lifts of the leg that contract and release the muscles in quick succession. If you place the palm of your hand on your thigh, you'll feel the muscles working beneath it.
- Repeat 16 times.
- Bend your knee and return your foot to the floor.
- Repeat with the other leg.
- Repeat both sides one more time; you can increase repetitions when you feel ready.

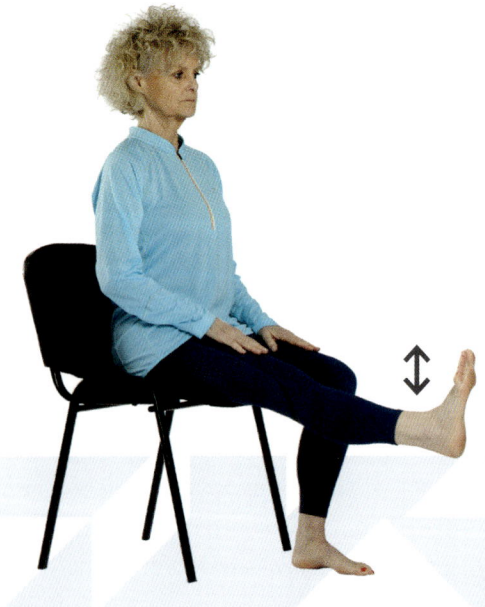

MIX AND MATCH LEG KICKS (I)

Benefits

For this exercise, you're going to challenge your coordination by combining both the knee lifts and the leg extension exercise together. Once again this will help strengthen your thigh muscles, which can boost knee stability, improve your posture and make walking easier, too.

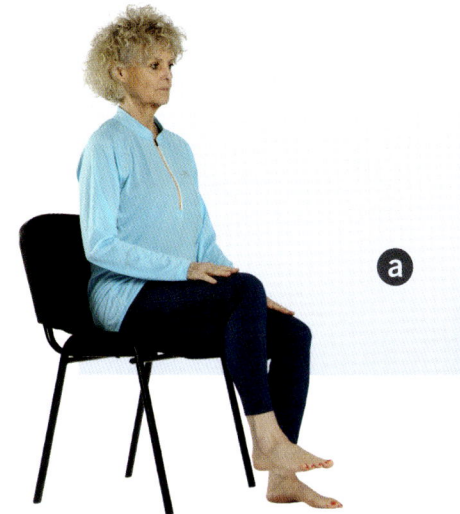

Method

- Sit up tall on your chair and move slightly forwards on your seat.
- Breathe in and as you breathe out lift your right foot off the floor keeping your knee bent at 90 degrees as you did for the knee lift exercise on page 99. **a**
- Breathe in again and as you breathe out lengthen and extend the leg out in front of you. **b**
- Breathe in as you hold the extended leg out in front of you and as you breathe out return the leg to the bent position and your foot to the floor.
- Repeat on the other leg.
- Complete 4 repetitions in total on each side and then if you're happy with how that feels, progress to 8 repetitions on each side.

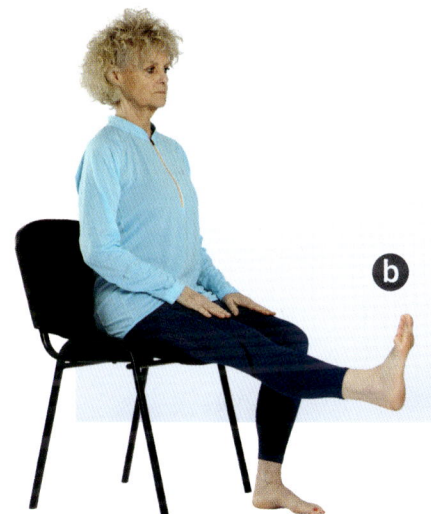

KNEE TO ELBOW ROTATION (1)

Benefits

This exercise will introduce a rotational movement to the mobility and coordination of the previous exercise and will also work your abdominal muscles, particularly your obliques (waist muscles).

Method

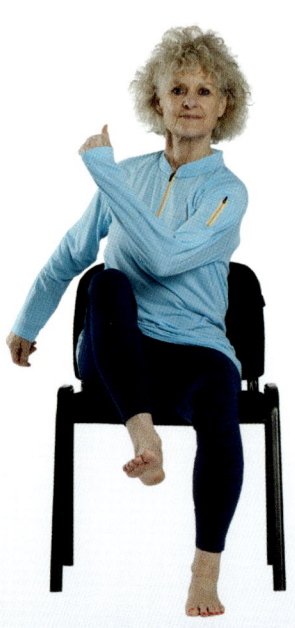

- Sit up tall on your chair.
- Take a breath in and as you breathe out, raise your right knee up to a 90-degree angle. At the same time rotate your torso towards it, bending your left elbow and lowering your arm and elbow towards the elevated right knee.
- Breathe in as you hold for a beat and as you breathe out return your leg and arm to the start position.
- If you can't touch your knee with your elbow, it doesn't matter. Just move towards it, gently twisting your torso, and don't force anything.
- Complete 4 repetitions on each side; increase the repetitions when you feel ready.
- If you find it easier, perform the exercise alternating between the sides.

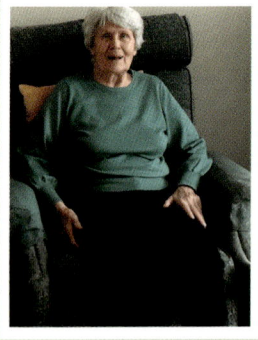

CASE STUDY

HAZEL BARNARD
AGE 84

'I swim once a week and was active until I fell a couple of months ago and hurt my knee, although it's definitely getting better and the chair exercises help. They help particularly with getting up out of a chair; I still need to ease myself up, but I can see the difference and I'm getting stronger and so is my leg.'

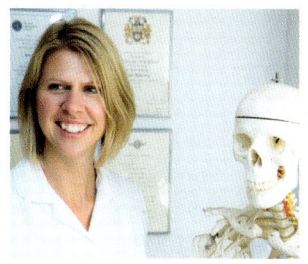

PROFESSIONAL ADVICE

JANE KAUSHAL
OSTEOPATH

Jane says:

'We all have signs of wear and tear in our joints past the age of 25. This will continue through the rest of our lives – resistance is futile! But numerous studies show that a person's symptoms do not have a direct correlation to their scan findings. You can have two people with similar hip X-ray findings and one is in a lot of pain and the other is doing very nicely, thank you. The reason for this difference is the "context" of that hip and the health of the muscles and other joints that affect the area. If you keep strong and flexible with good balance, by practising exercises regularly, you are more likely to cope well with wear and tear and be able to do what you want to do, without pain, for longer.'

HIPS

If you have had a hip replacement, please omit the following exercises and/or take professional advice on the correct exercises that are safe to do post-operatively and in the future. Please read the physiotherapist's advice on page 40 for more information.

Benefits

As we age our joints can begin to wear down. To keep them healthy we need to perform low-impact exercises such as those in this book to keep the hips flexible and healthy so that we can continue to put our shoes and socks on without difficulty and move with ease. We need a good hip range of motion to do that. Stiffness in our joints and particularly our hips and knees can creep up on us, so keep them moving. You will find some more hip exercises later on page 136 that require you to use the chair as a prop, holding on to the back of it for balance as you stand.

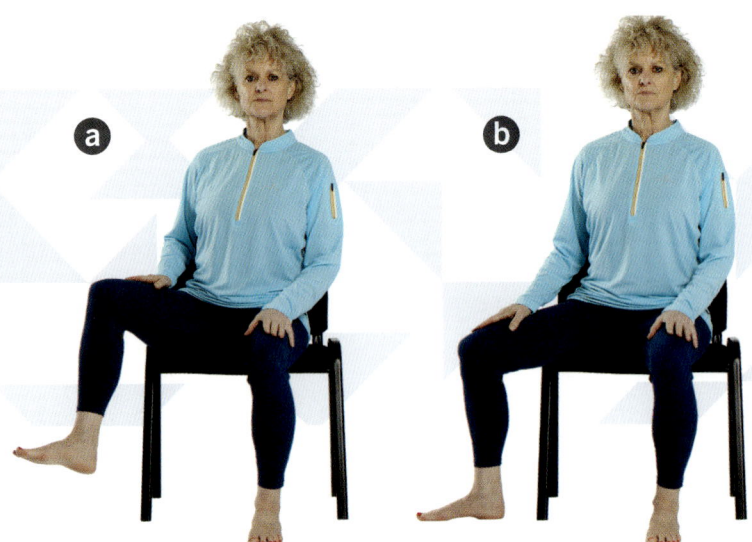

HIP OPENER (B)

Benefits

This is a great mobility exercise for your hips, improving flexibility and helping to maintain a good range of motion in the joint.

Method

- Sit up tall on your chair.
- Relax your shoulders and arms – you can place one hand on each thigh if you wish or keep them by your sides.
- Engage your abdominal muscles and/or your pelvic floor muscles.
- Breathe in and then as you breathe out, lift your right knee up to a 90-degree angle. (If you find it a challenge to lift your knee that high, then just lift to wherever is comfortable for you.)
- Keeping the movement flowing, open your hip out towards the right side of your chair, lifting your foot off the ground as if you're climbing over a small fence or getting out of a car. **a**
- Place your foot down on the floor to the right side of your chair. **b**
- Breathe in and as you breathe out lift the leg over the imaginary tiny fence and back to the front of your chair.
- Repeat on the other side.
- Repeat 4 times on each side.

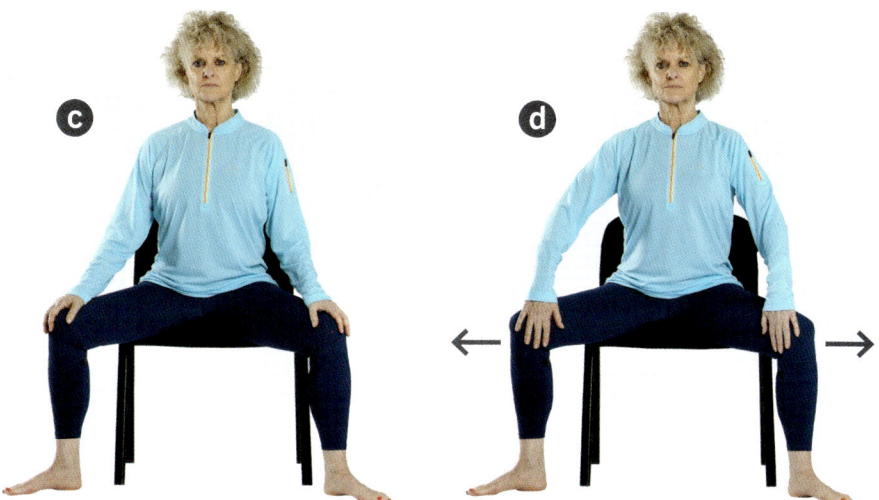

- When you've completed this exercise, move both legs out to the side of your chair. **c**
- Place your hands gently on the inside of both knees and pulse the legs in and out, creating small, fast movements back and forth so that you begin to feel a stretch on the inside of your thighs. **d**
- Repeat 8 times; increase the repetitions to 16 when you feel ready.
- Return your knees back to the front of your chair.

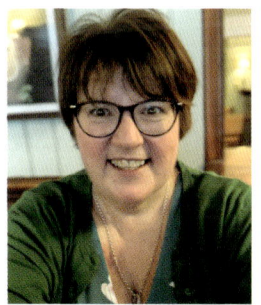

CASE STUDY

MOLLY FUCHS
AGE 58

'In 2020 I was diagnosed with stage 4 breast cancer, which is now incurable and in my pelvic bones. Harri's Chair Pilates and Yoga class helps me to keep exercising but at my own pace and at a level that I can manage, especially if I've just had treatment and it's one of my off days. I can still do lower leg exercises while seated (I used to be a runner) as well as the more traditional upper body exercises. But most importantly, I think the Chair Pilates and Yoga class has helped me not to feel different to anyone else.'

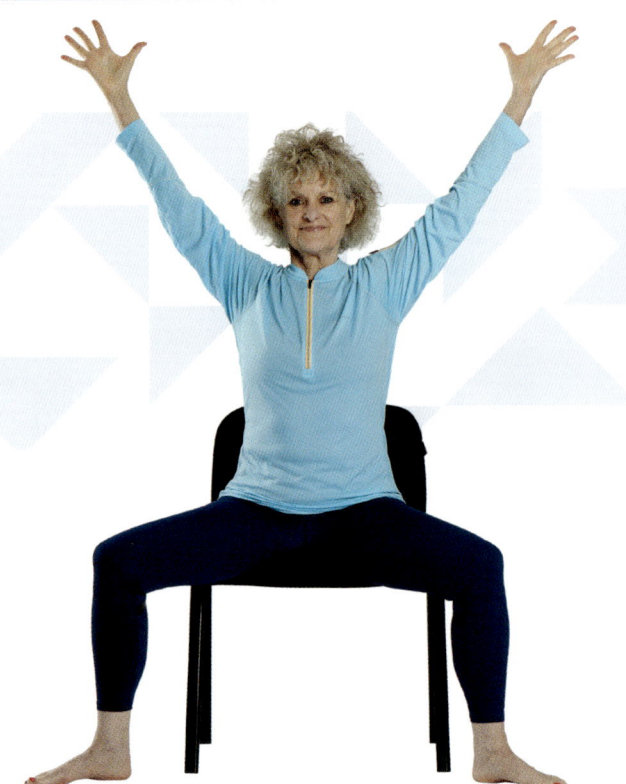

HIPPY HIPPY SHAKE (1)

Benefits

This is a coordination exercise that uses both legs and both arms at the same time. It is also quite an energising movement.

Method

- Sit up tall on your chair with your arms by your side.
- Take a breath in and as you breathe out, open your legs wide, knees still bent, to the side of your chair, and simultaneously extend both arms up in the air.
- Breathe in again as you hold the position for a beat.
- As you breathe out, return your arms and legs to the start position.
- Repeat 8 times, increasing the repetitions when you feel ready.
- If you prefer, you can perform this exercise more dynamically, breathing normally; it depends on how you're feeling and what your body is telling you to do.

CUSHION SQUEEZE (B)

Benefits

This exercise will work your inner thighs (adductors) and strengthen your knees and pelvic floor muscles. Having strong inner thighs will help stabilise your hips as you walk and go about your daily activities.

Method

- Grab a cushion, preferably one that is quite squishy so that it has some give, fold it in half and place it between your knees. If you own a small Pilates ball, you can use this instead of a cushion.
- Sit up tall on your chair.
- Breathe normally for this exercise and make sure you don't hold your breath as you concentrate on the movement.
- Give the cushion between your knees a good squeeze — you should feel your inner thigh muscles activate as you do this.
- Gently pulse — small squeezes, one after the other — for 8 repetitions.
- Hold the cushion tight between your knees after you have completed your 8 pulses.
- Pull up your pelvic floor muscles for a silent count of four as you continue to keep the cushion squeezed tightly between your knees, and then release.
- Repeat the 8 pulses and then hold once more.
- Repeat for 4 rounds.

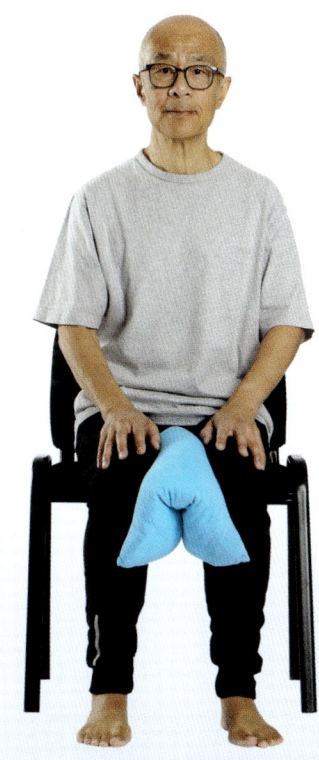

FEET SHUFFLE (B)

Benefits

This exercise is a simple coordination exercise that will also improve the flexibility of the feet and hips.

Method

- Sit up tall on your chair, take your feet wide, knees out to the side, lengthen through the spine.
- Engage your abdominal muscles and/or pelvic floor muscles.
- Slowly walk your feet back towards the front of your chair, swivelling them, heel to toe, heel to toe, sliding your feet across the floor until they are back in front of your chair.
- Repeat, going the other way, swivelling them outwards back towards the sides of your chair.
- Repeat 4 times and finish with your feet back in front of you.

First you are young; then you are middle-aged; then you are old; then you are wonderful.'

Lady Diana Cooper

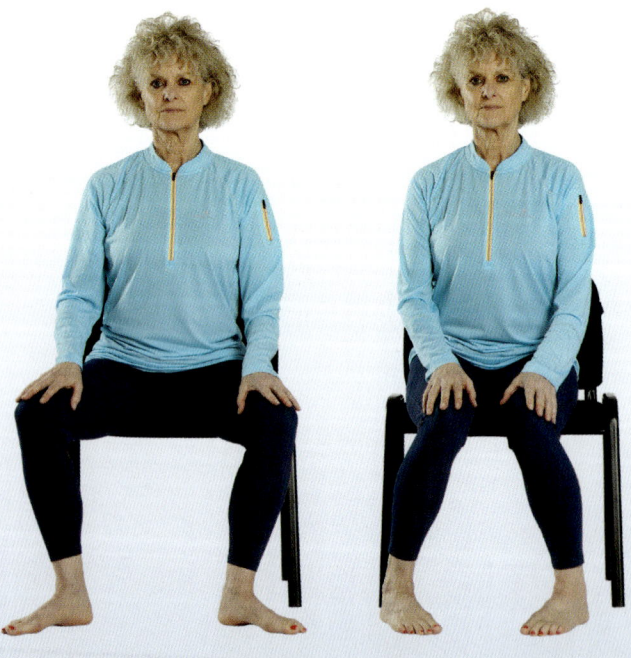

CROSS LEGS (I)

Benefits

It's never particularly good to sit with your legs crossed because it can lead to poor posture due to the misaligned way we tend to sit in this position.

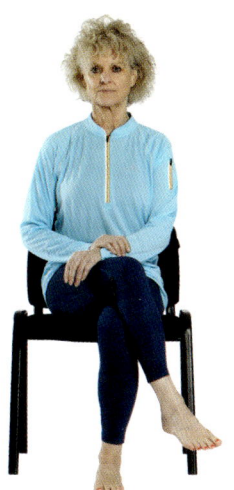

But for the purpose of this exercise, that is what we're going to do – cross our legs – but dynamically, and they won't stay crossed for long. This movement can improve flexibility and coordination, but if you have hip problems or have had a hip replacement, please omit this exercise and/or take advice from a health professional on the correct exercises to improve your range of movement and strength in that area.

Method

- Sit up tall on your chair.
- Take a breath in and as you breathe out, lift your right leg up and over your left thigh so that your legs are crossed.
- Breathe in again as you hold for a beat.
- As you breathe out, uncross the legs.
- Breathe in again and as you breathe out cross your left leg over your right thigh.
- Continue, alternating legs a few more times, speeding the movement up if you feel comfortable to do so.

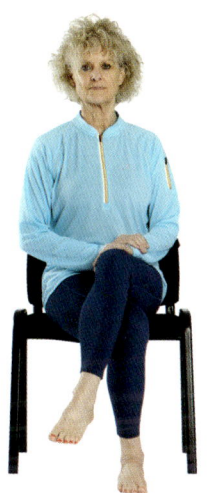

If this is challenging for you, cross your ankles instead.

- Extend your legs out in front of your chair and place one ankle over the top of the other.
- Repeat with the other ankle, taking turns to cross over each in turn.

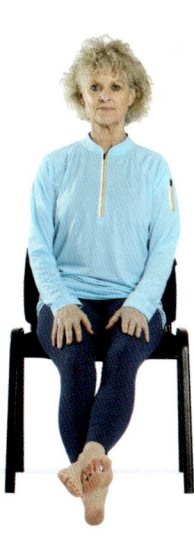

ABS AND LEGS COMBINED (I)

This exercise is more dynamic than most and can be performed slowly or faster depending on how you feel.

Benefits

As well as working your leg muscles and mobilising joints, you'll find that your abdominal muscles will engage as you perform this exercise, which is an added bonus.

Method

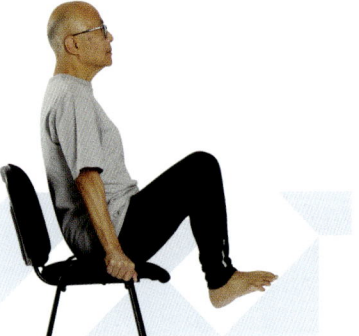

- Sit up tall and shift to the edge of your chair.
- Place the palms of your hands on either side beside your hips on your chair to anchor yourself.
- Breathe in, and as you breathe out, raise both your legs off the floor bringing your knees towards your torso. **a**
- Breathe in again as you hold for a beat.
- As you breathe out, return your feet to the floor.
- Repeat 4 times, increasing the repetitions when you feel ready.

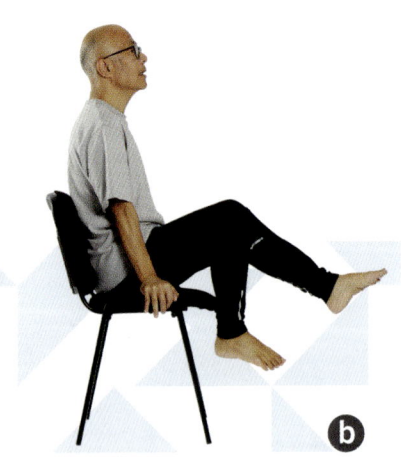

- Now, breathing normally, lift legs off the floor again.
- This time cycle your legs slowly forwards, lifting your knees up each time. **b**
- Aim for 8 cycles in one direction.
- Reverse the action, cycling backwards 8 times, resting in between if you feel you need to. As you begin to feel fitter you might like to increase the cycling repetitions.
- Remember to keep breathing as you might find yourself holding your breath as you concentrate.

CHAPTER 14

FEET, TOES AND ANKLES

When planning a regular exercise routine, feet strengthening and stretching exercises are probably not one of the first things you think to include. But keeping our feet healthy and happy as we age is just as important as keeping the rest of our body fit, well and strong. Our feet receive a huge amount of impact when we walk about and they also play an important part in our balance, which, of course, as already stated several times, can become more challenging as we age. Due to reduced levels of collagen, the fatty pads of our feet lose their cushioning and our feet can become weak or rigid if we do nothing to maintain our foot health.

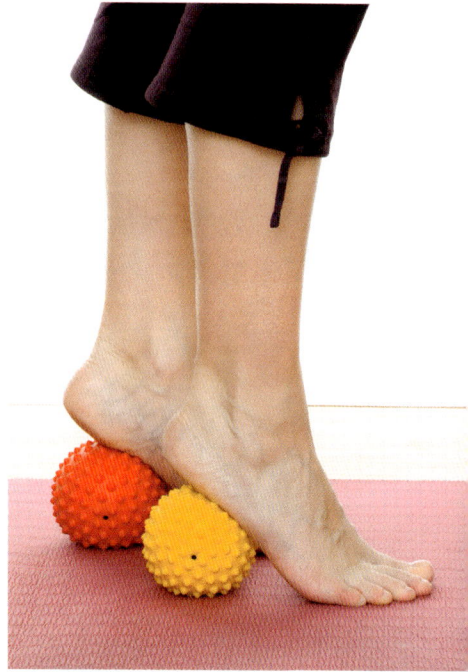

Benefits

By exercising our feet, toes and ankles regularly, we can improve circulation and muscle mass, just like exercise does for the rest of the body. I cover balance exercises later on (*see* p. 132), but by adding the following feet, toe and ankle movements into your daily routine, you'll find that not only will they become stronger but your balance will improve as well.

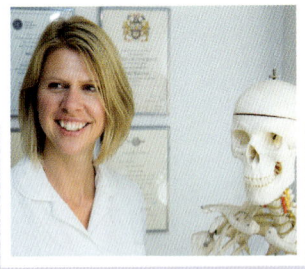

OSTEOPATH, JANE KAUSHAL

Jane says:

'"Use it or lose it" is even more relevant when it comes to foot flexibility and health in later life. After the age of 60 many people's feet become stiff or even rigid if they do nothing to maintain mechanical foot health. Rigid feet do not balance properly, as they can't adapt to the surface they are on, and the intrinsic muscles within the feet become very weak. Feet are therefore at the mercy of external forces and can make bunion deformities or plantar fascia pain more likely to develop. Any balancing and stretching exercise with bare feet is helpful, and Pilates is ideal. It will move the feet and ankles through a full range of movement and maintain the strength of the small muscles deep in the feet. In addition, I would recommend standing on one foot when you brush your teeth – left foot in the morning and the other foot before you go right to bed!'

FOOT PEDALLING (B)

The Achilles tendon stretches from the bone of your heel at the back of your leg to your calf muscles that sit just above it. Traditionally in a Pilates class, these exercises are performed standing up, but like many of the exercises in this book, we can benefit just as much from performing them while sitting down.

Benefits

Along with our feet, our calf muscles can become quite tight and stiff, especially if they're not used much, so stretching and strengthening them is vital to keeping them healthy and preventing injury.

Method

- Sit up tall on your chair and breathe normally.
- Alternating the feet, begin by coming up and down on the balls of your feet, raising each heel in turn and then gently placing it back down on the floor.
- Perform 16 repetitions.

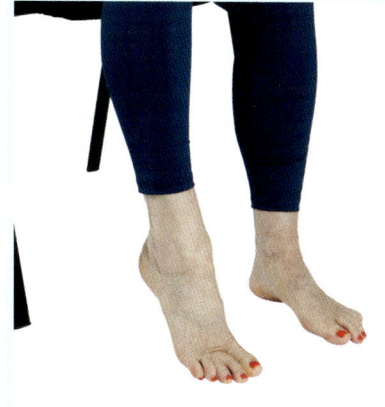

- Now come up on to the balls of both feet at the same time.
- Stay there for a beat, feeling the stretch in the sole of your foot and your calf muscles (at the back of your leg) activating.
- With control, lower your heels to the ground as slowly as you can.
- Repeat 4 times.

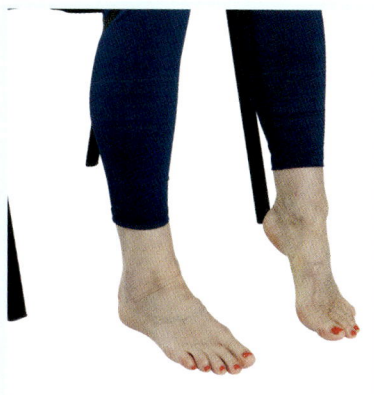

- Follow this with some fast up-and-down heel raises with both feet at the same time. Perform 16 repetitions.
- Now place your heels together and turn your toes out to a ten to two position.
- Raise your heels up and down: gently raise up on to the balls of your feet and then lower your heels down to the floor again.

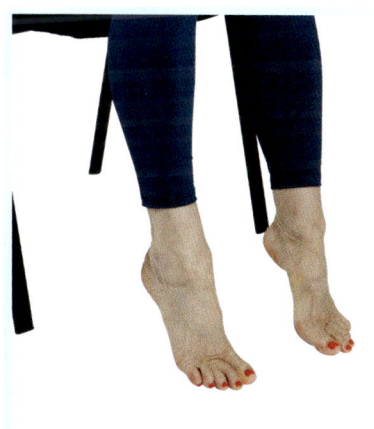

BRAIN GYM FOR FEET (B)

Benefits

This simple exercise will not only stretch and strengthen the feet but also challenge your coordination and concentration.

Method

- Sit up tall on your chair and breathe normally.
- Place your hands, palm down on your thighs and relax your shoulders.
- Rise up on to the ball of your right foot only. **a**
- Now rise up on to the ball of your left foot — so both heels are now raised. **b**
- Take your right heel slowly down to the floor. **c**
- Take your left heel down to the floor.
- Repeat the moves, alternating right, left, right, left, 4 times.
- Change sides and repeat, starting with the left foot.

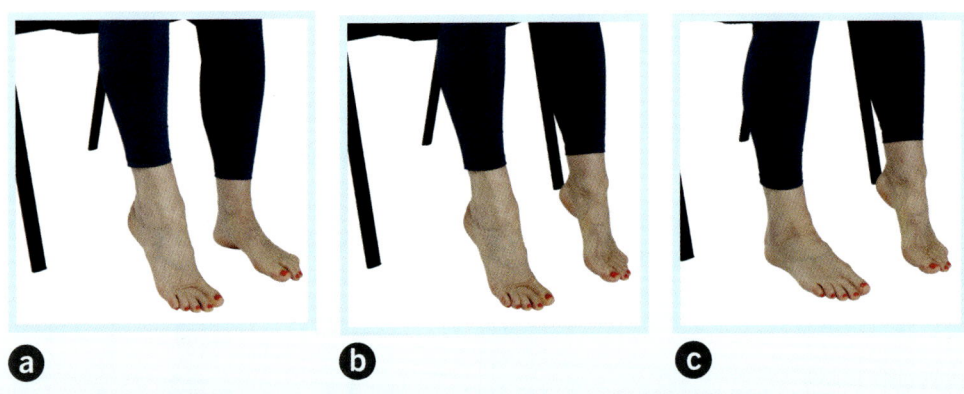

a   **b**   **c**

TOES

Benefits

The following toe exercises — which you will need to perform with bare feet — will strengthen and improve the mobility of the toes and inner foot muscles, stretch the arches and improve overall coordination and blood flow. If you have overlapping toes, blisters, corns, bunions or any other condition affecting your feet, this can have a huge impact on the rest of your body. Once you've had a go at the following exercises, and if you would like to try something a bit more challenging but ultimately very beneficial for the feet, have a go at Toe Yoga at the end of this section (*see* p. 120).

SPLAY YOUR TOES (B)

Benefits

When your toes are splayed it can benefit your whole body and even impact your ankles, knees and lower back. Practising splaying your toes regularly will improve your balance and general stability, and increase blood flow to the toes, especially if your footwear is tight or your feet swell.

Method

- Place your feet parallel and visible to you when you look down at them on the floor and spread your toes as wide as you possibly can. This might not be far, and to begin with, if they need some help, use your fingers to guide them apart. Alternatively, you may find you have quite a lot of movement.
- Hold the toe stretch for a silent count of four and then release.
- Repeat 4 times.

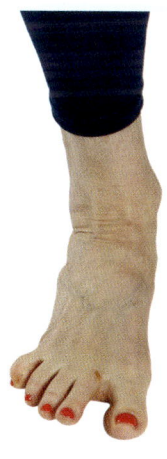
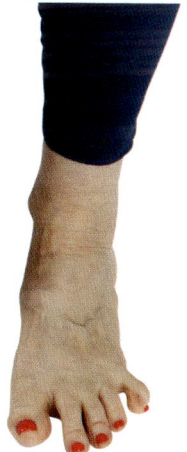

BIG TOE STRETCH (B)

Benefits

Like the rest of the foot, we need to keep a healthy range of movement in our big toes. This is also a good exercise to do if you've been on your feet all day or wearing tight shoes.

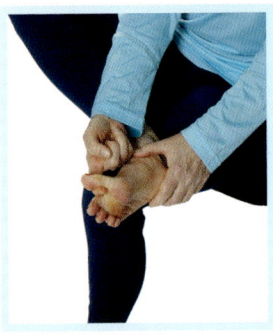

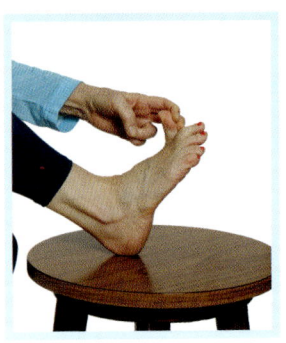

Method

- Sit up tall on your chair.
- Raise your right foot and rest it on your left thigh.
- With your fingers, gently stretch your big toe up and down and from side to side.
- Now repeat, holding each position for the silent count of four.
- Repeat on your other foot.
- If it's a struggle to place your right foot on your left thigh, bend down to your toe while sitting on your chair and perform the exercise that way.
- If that's not possible, find another chair and place it in front of the one you're sitting on (or use your coffee table), bend your knee and place your foot on its seat (or table top), which should make it easier to reach.

CASE STUDY

BETTY BAKER
AGE 89

'Chair exercises are good for you at our age and I would do more, but I have osteoarthritis in my knee, which is painful, but I know I need to keep it moving. Sit to stand is hard; I can go a little way at a time and then I sit and rest. I've just got to keep at it so that I can keep mobile for as long as possible, but the feet and ankle exercises are a good start.'

TOE CURLS (B)

Benefits

Toe curls can improve the overall strength of your feet and increase blood flow. This is also a coordination exercise.

Method

- Grab a tea towel or small hand towel and place it beneath one foot. **ⓐ**
- Sit up tall on your chair. Have the heel of the foot that's placed on the tea towel near the edge.
- Lift all your toes of that foot up off the floor.
- Hold for a silent count of four.
- Now fold your toes in the opposite direction with the aim of picking the tea towel up with your folded toes (the coordination bit!) and moving it towards your chair using your toes — you're not using your whole foot, just your toes as you pull the towel closer.
- Repeat on the other side. **ⓑ**

- Be aware of what the rest of your body is doing at the same time — are you holding your breath? Are you clenching your fists or your jaw? Are your shoulders relaxed or are they up around your ears?
- Concentration can cause tension in the rest of the body, so try and stay relaxed and be body aware — only one foot should be moving at a time.

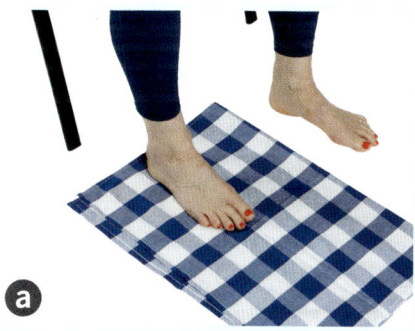

ⓐ

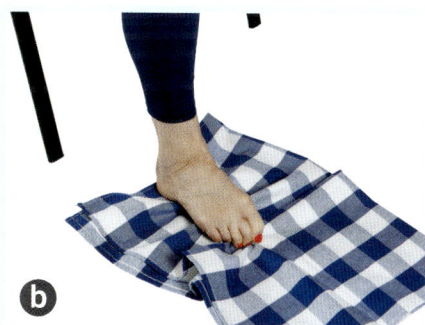

ⓑ

TOE YOGA (I)

Benefits

Yes, this really is a thing! And quite challenging. But strong toes can promote good balance, posture and support for the body as already stated in the preceding exercises, so have a go.

For this exercise, you are going to isolate just your big toes – you might like to do the big toe stretch on page 118 first if you haven't already.

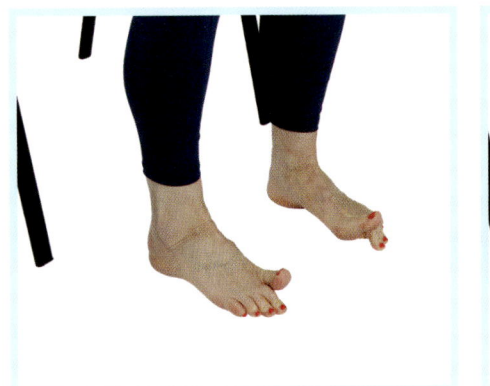 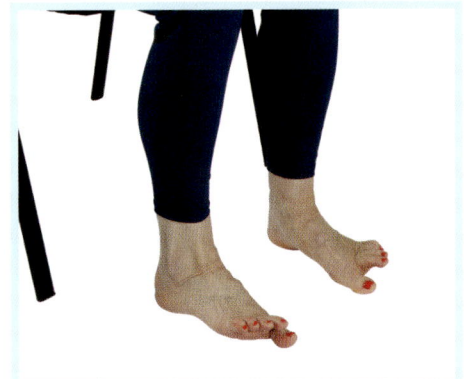

Method

- Sit up tall on your chair. Make sure your feet are visible to you below your knees as you look down at the floor.
- Try to lift both your big toes off the floor, leaving the other toes on the ground.
- Hold for a silent count of four and then release.
- Repeat 4 more times.
- Now, for the next part of this exercise, keep your big toes on the ground and lift the other four toes on your foot.
- Hold for a silent count of four and then release.
- Repeat 4 more times.
- With practice, this gets easier! If you want to challenge your feet further, try isolating each toe in turn to create a Mexican wave!

ANKLE MOBILITY (B)

Benefits

This is a simple but important exercise to achieve and maintain full range of movement and improve strength in the ankles and feet. Not only your feet but also your ankles have to withstand the impact of walking or standing and this exercise will help them do so. The pointing and flexing of the foot improves flexibility and strengthens and lengthens the muscles of the front and back leg.

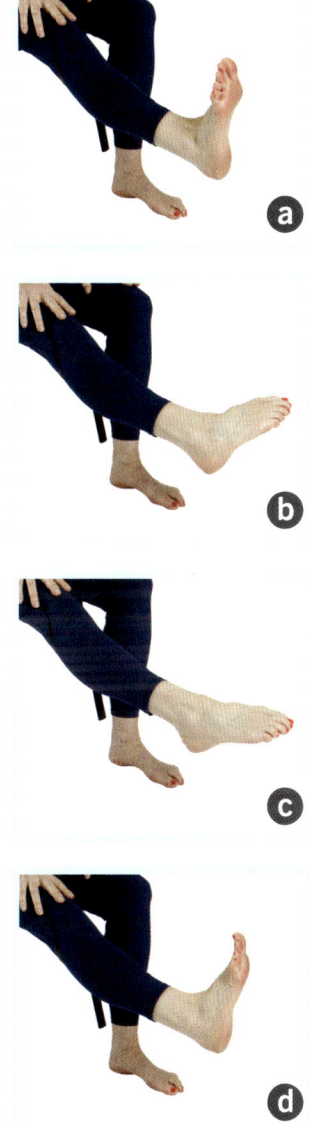

Method

- Sit up tall on your chair and rest the palms of your hands on your thighs.
- Raise your right leg and extend it out in front of you. **a**
- If you find it hard to extend and keep your leg in that position for any length of time, hold your leg – place your hands under your thigh so that you are supporting your leg.
- Rotate your ankle very slowly in one direction 4 times. **b**
- Reverse the movement, rotating in the other direction.
- Try and draw a full circle with your toes when rotating your ankle, keeping your knee and lower leg stable; try not to let that part of your leg join in.
- Return your foot to centre.
- Alternate pointing **c** and flexing **d** (when your toes are pointed upwards) your toes 4 times on each foot.
- Be aware of what the rest of your body is doing. Sometimes it joins in and you might find your head moving around in the same direction as your foot! Try and stay relaxed.

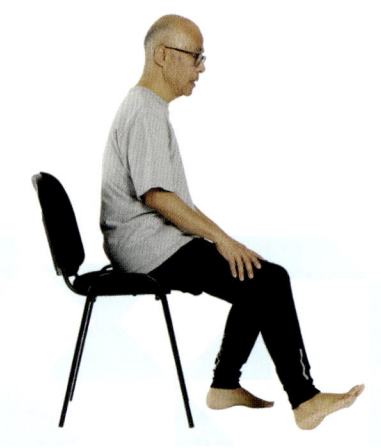

WRITE YOUR NAME (I)

Benefits

As an extension to the ankle mobility exercises on page 121, now you are going to write your name with your toes and then your heel. This is also a coordination exercise.

Method

- Sit up tall on your chair.
- Lift your right foot off the ground; support your leg if you need to by placing your hands underneath your thigh, or extend the leg out in front of you.
- Write your name in the air with your toes.
- Repeat on the other side.
- Now write your name with your heel on the ground, foot flexed.

FOOT MASSAGE (B)

For this exercise, you'll need a tennis ball or a small massage ball (one with spikes is best).

Benefits

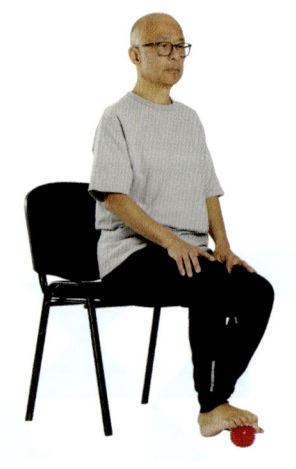

If you spend a lot of time on your feet, they can become tired, achy and sore. So what's better than a foot massage? Massaging your feet can relieve and reduce discomfort in the arch of the foot and ease the pain associated with plantar fasciitis.

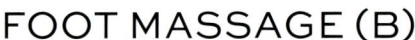

Method

- Sitting on your chair, place the ball or massager under the sole of your right foot.
- Sit up tall on your chair, lengthen through the spine and keep your shoulders relaxed.
- Roll the ball back and forth, from toe to heel, for about a minute, applying as much pressure as you can but making sure it's comfortable.
- Now rotate the ball first one way and then the other way, round and round in circles on the sole of your foot.
- Repeat several times.

- If you find an especially sore spot, keep going and concentrate the pressure on that area.
- Don't forget to do the other foot!

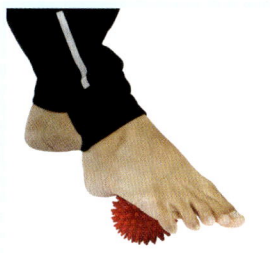

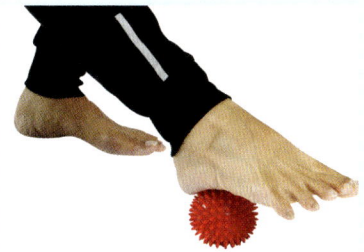

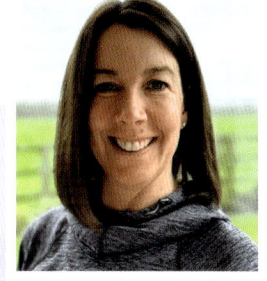

PROFESSIONAL ADVICE

SARA CARTER
PHYSIOTHERAPIST

Sara who works with older adults says: 'Osteoarthritis is the most common form of arthritis. Common symptoms include pain and reduced movement in the joint. Exercise is important for people with arthritis, it increases strength and flexibility and can also reduce pain. If you have stiff, painful joints, the thought of exercise can be overwhelming, therefore finding an exercise programme that allows you to start moving in a manageable way is important. Exercise strengthens the muscles that surround the joints giving them more protection and reducing the stress on the joints. Lack of exercise makes the joints more stiff and painful. Any movement no matter how small can help. If you have not exercised for a while, starting slowly to ease your joints into movement is important and therefore something such as chair-based Pilates and yoga, which are low impact, helps keep the joint stress low.'

CHAPTER 15

FACIAL EXERCISES

Like toe yoga, face yoga is also a thing! Any internet search will produce the promise that facial yoga or facial exercises can reduce fine lines, sagging skin and help to make us look younger.

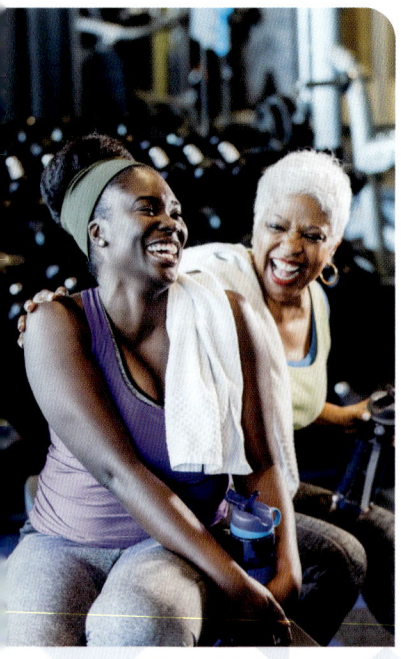

Personally, I am not convinced, but like the rest of our body, our facial muscles can definitely benefit from being exercised and this can boost our complexions, brighten up a tired face, de-stress and generally make us feel better about ourselves.

However, a research paper entitled 'Association of Facial Exercise with the Appearance of Ageing' published by the *National Institute of Health* in 2018 concluded that facial exercises can indeed go some way to improving our facial appearance. Additionally, it is well documented that massaging your face can improve blood flow, stimulate circulation and reduce puffiness. So here are a few facial exercises for you to try.

MOUTH

Benefits

Apart from the fact that smiling automatically makes us feel brighter, this exercise will help relax the muscles around your cheeks and mouth. If you tend to clench your teeth and jaw or hold tension in this area of your face, particularly when you're concentrating hard on something, give this exercise a go and see how it makes you feel.

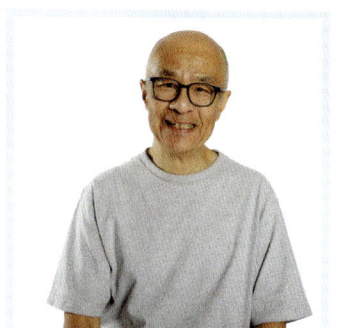

Method

- Simply smile the widest smile you possibly can.
- Hold the exaggerated smile for a beat and then move your mouth in the opposite direction and purse your lips as if you are about to plant a big kiss on someone's cheek.
- Try not to hold your breath.
- Repeat 10 times.

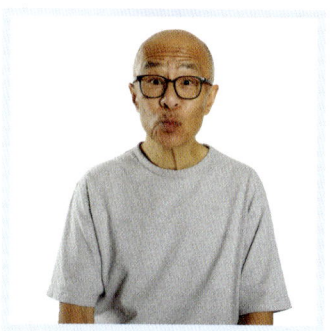

CHEEKS

Benefits

As we age our facial muscles, and specifically our cheeks, can take on a hollow look. This exercise will help add colour to your cheeks and exercise the muscles in the area in the hope of preventing this.

Method

- Take a big breath in.
- As you breathe out, puff out your cheeks as if you are blowing up a balloon, but keep your lips relaxed. Hold for a beat before releasing.
- Repeat 4 times.

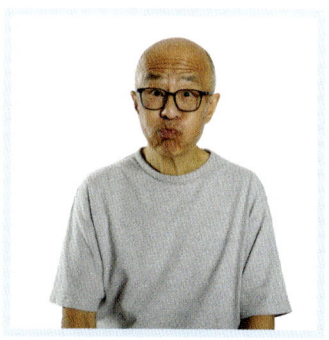

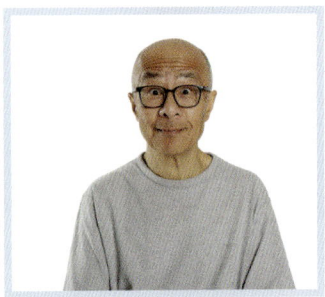

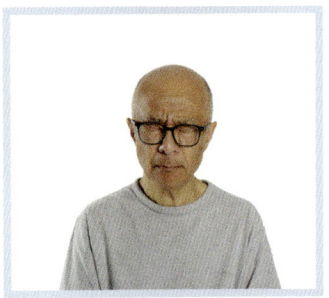

EYES

Benefits

This exercise works the muscles around the eyes and forehead; if your eyes feel heavy and tired, this can go some way towards waking them (and you!) up.

Method

- Open your eyes as wide as you can and hold for a silent count of four.
- Then squeeze them shut tight — you'll find that the rest of your face tightens up, too.
- Release all the muscles.
- Check that you're not clenching your jaw and then repeat the exercise 4 more times.

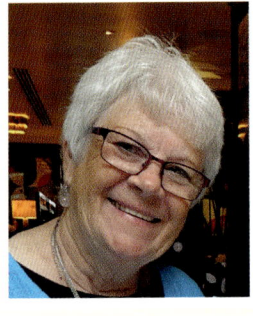

CASE STUDY

BARBARA MURFITT
AGE 75

'Since practising these seated exercises I've increased the mobility in my stiff joints — especially in my arthritic shoulder joint — and overall, I've gained strength. Mat Pilates was difficult for me as I was unable to get down or up without help and so chair exercises have been brilliant. The sit-to-stand [see p.128] exercise has definitely increased the strength in my legs and lower back, and the hand and feet exercises and stretches have given me so much more freedom of movement. The balance exercise, holding on to the back of the chair at the end of the session, is so good for me — slowly but surely I have gained good balance on one leg and this gives such a sense of achievement. Not only do we have fun, encouragement and group support in the class, but Chair Pilates and Yoga leaves me with a feeling of peace and an overall sense of well-being.'

CHAPTER 16

SIT TO STAND

Moving from sitting to standing strengthens the muscles in your thighs and core, including your back and glutes (buttocks). More importantly, it's really useful to do if you've had knee or hip surgery, but please take advice from your doctor or physical therapist about when it would be appropriate to start these exercises. (See the physiotherapist advice on page 40.) This movement is so important to us as we age to improve, or sustain, our ability to get up out of a chair with ease, or get out of a car, or not get stuck on the loo!

Based on your current ability, this chapter features a few variations for you to try. If you struggle to get up off your chair, then start with the version marked **(B)** for beginner; once you feel confident and stronger, you can work your way through the other versions. If, on the other hand, you have no problem standing from a seated position but would like to improve your strength and maintain it, start with one of the later versions.

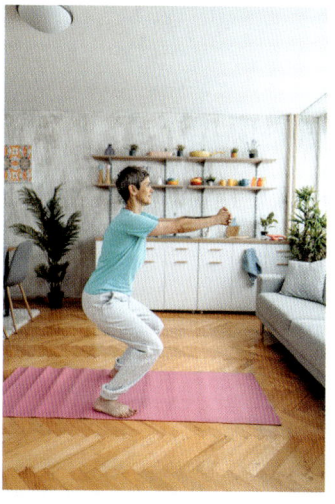

Note: If you're worried that the chair might move or you'll miss the seat of the chair as you sit, have your calf muscles (back of your lower legs) touching the chair slightly as you stand up; that way you'll know you're safe and that the chair is there.

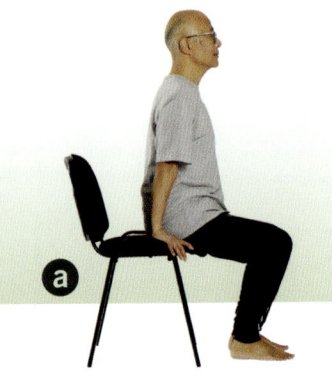

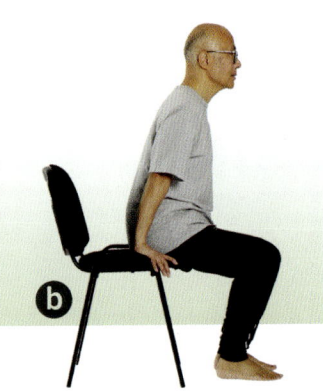

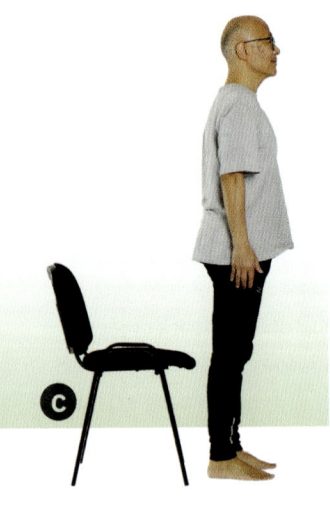

MOVING FROM SITTING TO A STANDING POSITION

Benefits

This sit-to-stand movement can make a huge difference to our everyday life if we practise it daily, as we need to keep this important function going so that we can remain independent and ward off frailty. Sitting for long periods of time can weaken the muscles that are used in this exercise, which means you are more likely to injure yourself or fall.

Method

Depending on your ability and mobility, you can use your arms to lever yourself up off the chair (B), take your arms in front of your torso and clasp your hands together (I), or raise your arms above your head as you stand, which is more challenging.

Version 1 (B)

- Sit slightly forwards, towards the edge of your chair, your feet placed firmly on the ground, hip-width apart below your knees.
- Place your hands on either side of your hips on your chair, palms down. **a**
- Engage your abdominal muscles.
- Take a breath in and as you breathe out, tilt yourself slightly forwards and lift yourself off the chair, using your hands to lever yourself up if you need to. **b**
- Breathe in as you stand tall, lengthening through your spine. **c**
- Take a moment here and then as you breathe out, bend your knees a little and push your hips out behind you as you slowly sit back down again.

- Repeat 8 times, take a breather and repeat. But if this is really challenging, start with 2–3 repetitions and leave it there.
- Keep practising and eventually you'll find you can comfortably manage 8 repetitions and more. As you get stronger, you'll find you won't need to lever yourself up off the chair any more.

Version 2 (I)

- Sit towards the edge of your chair, your feet placed firmly on the ground, hip-width apart below your knees.
- Extend your arms out in front of you and clasp your hands together. Or, if you prefer, cross your arms over your chest. Ⓐ
- Engage your abdominal muscles.
- Take a breath in and as you breathe out, tilt yourself slightly forwards and lift yourself up off the chair. Ⓑ
- Breathe in while you stand for a moment. Ⓒ
- As you breathe out, bend your knees a little and push your hips out behind you as you slowly sit back down, keeping your arms extended out in front of you.
- Repeat 8 times, increasing the repetitions when you feel more confident. The more you do, the stronger you will become.

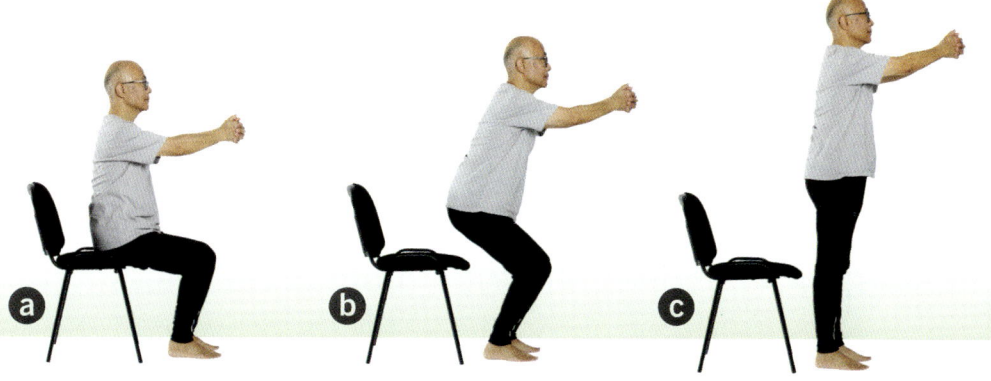

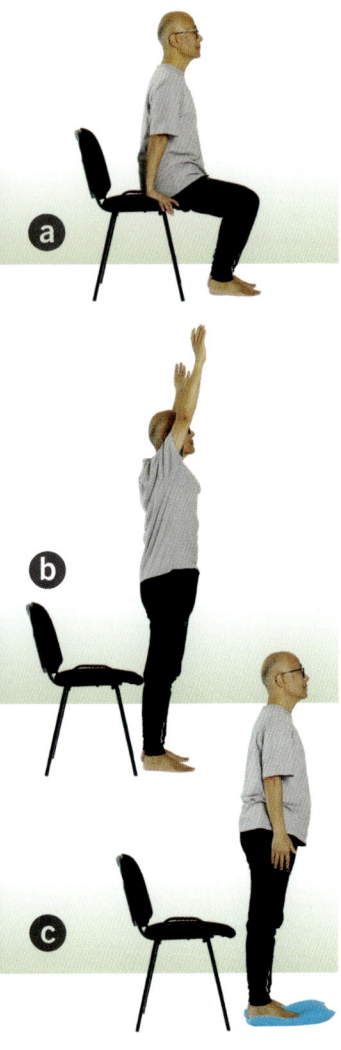

Version 3

This version of the sit-to-stand exercise is for when you feel you are ready for something a bit more challenging. But please make sure, before you attempt either of the following suggestions, that you are already comfortable with Version 2.

- Sit slightly forwards on your chair with your feet placed firmly on the ground hip-width apart below your knees. **a**
- Engage your abdominal muscles.
- Take a breath in and as you breathe out, tilt yourself slightly forwards and lift yourself up off the chair, while raising your arms above your head at the same time. **b**
- Breathe in as you stand tall, lengthening through your spine.
- As you breathe out, bend your knees a little and push your hips out behind you as you slowly sit back down, returning your arms to your sides.

- Finally, to challenge your balance, place a flattish pillow underneath your feet so that when you stand up you have to balance on something a little uneven as well. But before you do, make sure that you can comfortably complete all the versions of the sit-to-stand exercise and that your balance is sound. **c**

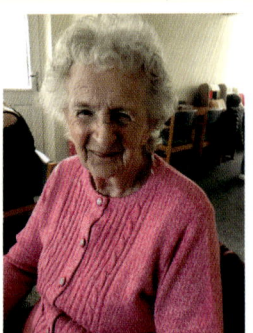

CASE STUDY

JOAN DUNNE
AGE 87

'Sometimes I feel like a tin man! My daughter and granddaughter nag me to keep my posture straight and these chair exercises help me a lot. I find getting out of my daughter's car awkward as one of my legs is better than the other, so these sit-to-stand movements help that. The neck exercises help the stiffness in my neck, too, and I do them regularly.'

HALFWAY SIT TO STAND (1)

Benefits

This is an adaptation of a recognisable yoga posture that, just like the sit-to-stand movement on page 128, strengthens your legs, your back, your hips and your buttocks. The yoga posture is coincidentally called 'chair'. If you lift your arms at the same time, then your shoulders will work as well, and to a certain extent, this exercise can challenge your balance. Basically, you will perform the sit-to-stand exercise but only go halfway back down to the chair, stopping mid-air and holding the pose.

Method

- Sit slightly forwards on your chair with your feet placed firmly on the ground hip-width apart below your knees.
- Breathe in, and as you breathe out lift yourself up as if standing, but stop halfway, raising your arms in the air.
- Hold for a silent count of four, making sure that you're not holding your breath.
- Take another breath in, then breathe out as you sit back down on the chair.

- Experiment with this posture by holding different levels of the stand but know that the chair is behind you should you need to sit down quickly.
- Practise this a couple of times. If you find that raising your arms at the same time is too much, then keep them by your side or just raise them a little way to begin with.

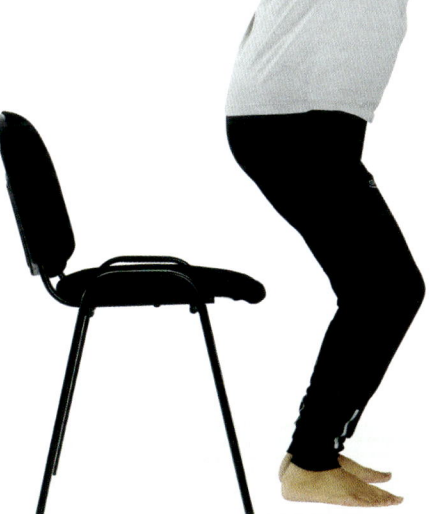

CHAPTER 17

BALANCE EXERCISES

You're now going to use the chair as a prop to practise balancing. As already stated numerous times earlier in the book, as we age our ability to balance sadly declines. To prevent falls and to maintain good balance, we need to have good proprioception, coordination and strong ankles and feet.

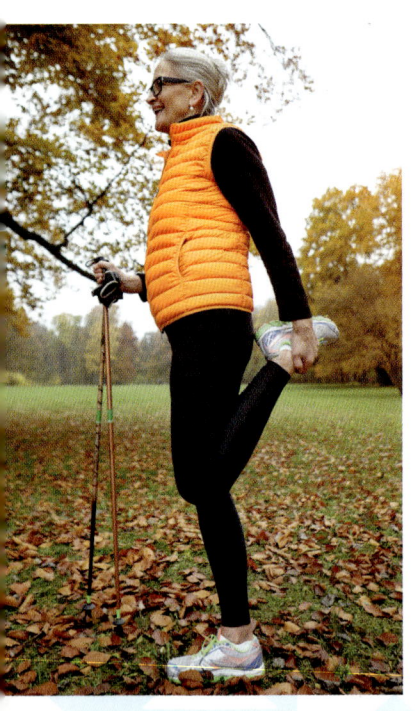

By practising balance, you will help the brain to recognise and cope with changes in terrain when you walk. The exercises will also help with concentration. You might find that as you practise these exercises you discover that your balance is better on one side of your body than the other; this is quite normal. Not only are falls more likely as we age, which, of course, can lead to injuries, but we become understandably anxious about falling and this, believe it or not, can make matters worse. Consequently, this fear of falling can prevent us from doing the things we love to do, like going out and socialising or taking walks, and once this happens, a downward spiral of frailty occurs both mentally and physically.

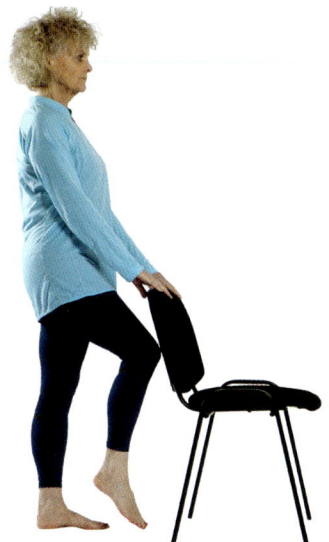

Life is like riding
a bicycle. To keep
your balance, you
must keep moving.'

Albert Einstein

You may find that on some days you can balance better than on other days. If you aren't sleeping well or are stressed, this will affect your ability to balance, so don't be disheartened; keep practising.

If you know you're wobbly and your balance isn't too good, or you're not sure and feel nervous, start with Balance 1 (B), below.

BALANCE 1 (B)

- Stand tall behind your chair and place both hands on the back of it.
- Breathing normally (you're likely to hold your breath here, so try and remember to breathe!) fix your gaze and concentrate on something ahead of you that's not moving.
- Take a moment to perform a few pelvic tilts and find your neutral spine (see p. 23).
- Raise your right leg, bending at the knee, just a little so that your toe is just off the ground.
- Hold the position, still holding on to the back of the chair, for a silent count of four.
- Place your foot back down on the floor.
- Repeat on the other side.

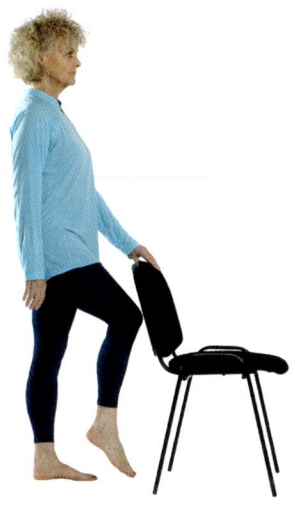

Note: If you're happy with your balance, try taking one hand away from the back of the chair and see what a difference this makes – please be careful and do this in stages so that you can monitor your balance ability. If you feel really wobbly, then keep both hands on the back of the chair.

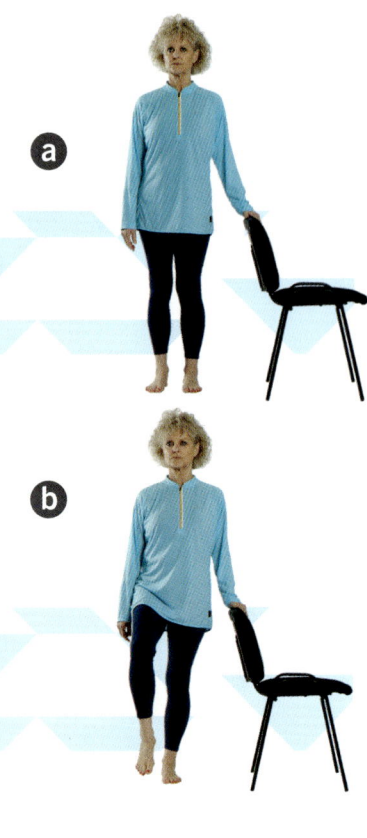

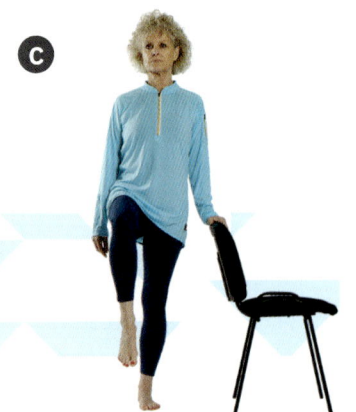

BALANCE 2 (B)

If you think you can balance but not for long, try this exercise.

- Stand beside your chair and hang on to the back of it with your left hand, with your right arm by your side. **a**
- Stand tall, and engage your abdominal muscles.
- Fix your gaze – concentrate on something ahead of you that isn't moving, as this will help you focus and balance.
- Breathe in and as you breathe out, slowly raise your right foot off the floor a little way. **b**
- Hold for a moment.
- Then replace your foot and repeat on the other side.

- Once you feel confident with this, progress to lifting your hand off the back of the chair: try lifting it off for a second or two.
- Let it hover over the back of the chair, then replace your hold. You'll find that your body will soon get the message and your balance will improve. But please take care.
- Try lifting your leg a little higher off the ground, if you feel confident. **c**
- Another way to help your balance is to touch the floor with your toe, then take your foot away and balance.
- Each time you wobble, return your toe back to the floor for a second.
- Repeat 4 times on each side.

There is no right or wrong way to go about this – we all have different levels of ability, but by practising we will improve our balance, which makes for safer walking and no falls.

BALANCE 3 (I)

Stand tall beside your chair in case you have a wobble and need to hold on to something – even if our balance is good, we all still wobble sometimes.

- Breathe in and as you breathe out, raise your right leg to a level that is comfortable for you; it doesn't have to be high.
- Keep standing tall and lengthened through your spine with your shoulders relaxed.
- Breathe in as you stand tall and as you breathe out, lift your left arm up in the air above your head while your right knee remains raised.
- Breathe in again and as you breathe out, lower your arm to your side, still keeping your leg raised.
- Repeat the arm sequence one more time, still standing on one leg.
- Change sides and repeat. Increase the repetitions when you feel more confident.

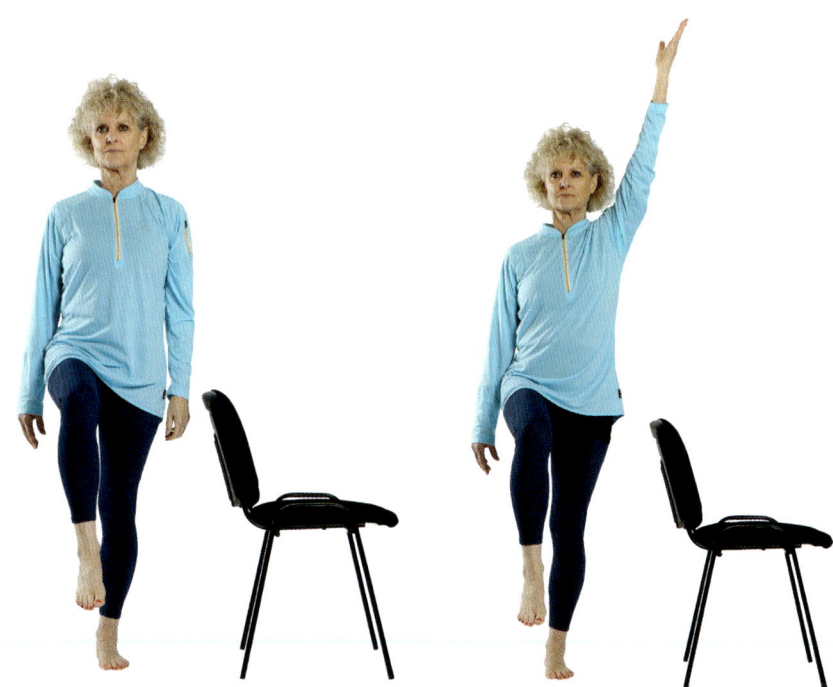

HIP OPENER BALANCE (I)

Benefits

This exercise once again uses the chair as a prop. This mobility exercise will really open up the hips, stretch your legs and challenge your balance. I suggest that this movement be practised very gently to begin with. It isn't suitable if you have serious hip or knee issues. Before you attempt the leg swings, please make sure you've tried some of the simpler exercises for the legs and the hips in this book (*see* p. 96) as a warm-up because you'll find that this is a more dynamic exercise than the ones performed while seated — the seated version of this exercise is on page 106. We're going to start with some gentle rotations of the hip, opening out the hip to the side and lifting the leg slightly as if climbing over a low stile.

Method

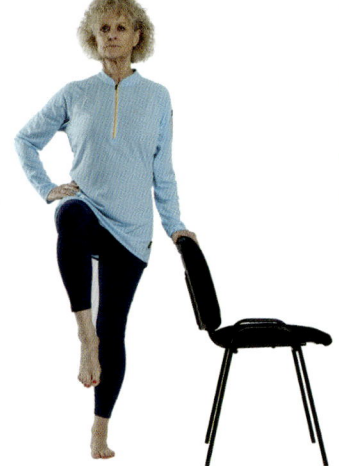

- Stand at the side of your chair, holding on to the back of it with one hand. Make sure you have space around you to move your leg backwards, forwards and out to the side.
- Try to keep a lengthened spine as you move your leg. It's easy to collapse in your centre and become slightly hunched, so make a conscious effort to keep upright and tall.
- Breathe in and as you breathe out, lift your leg up and circle your knee in an outwards motion to open out your hip and so that your leg rotates towards the side of your body.
- Breathe in again as you hold the knee to the side (you can put your toes down on the floor).
- As you breathe out, reverse the move and return your leg to the front.
- Repeat 4 times and then turn around and perform it on the other side.

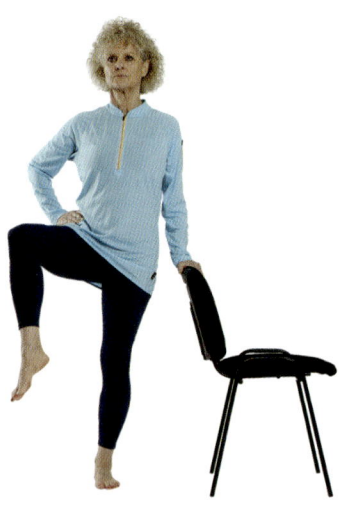

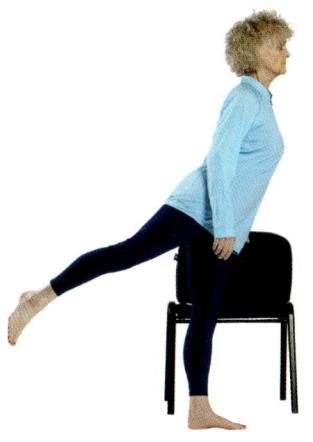 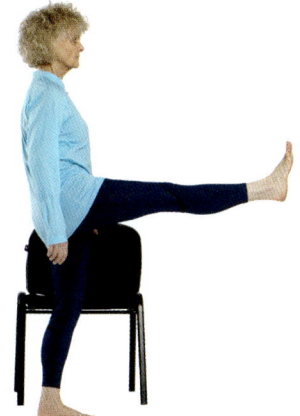

LEG SWING BALANCE (I)

Method

- Stand tall still holding on to the chair. Once again think about your posture, find your neutral spine (see p. 23) and keep your back lengthened, trying not to collapse in your centre.
- Breathe normally for this exercise.
- Gently swing one leg backwards and forwards – front to back, like a pendulum – not kicking but smooth, keeping the leg and movement relaxed and free. The swing should be low and comfortable.
- Repeat 4 times and then perform it on the other side.
- If this movement is comfortable and you find it easy, then you can add light ankle weights to your legs to make it more challenging and, later, increase the repetitions.

SQUAT (I)

Benefits

This is an excellent exercise to perform, as it strengthens hips and knee joints and lower body muscles. Very similar to the sit-to-stand exercise on page 128 and chair pose on page 131. The difference is that you don't get to sit down between each movement or at the end and the knee bend will be lower. If you have serious hip or knee problems or are post-operative, please check with your health professional that this exercise is suitable for you. See physiotherapist Sara Carter's advice on page 40.

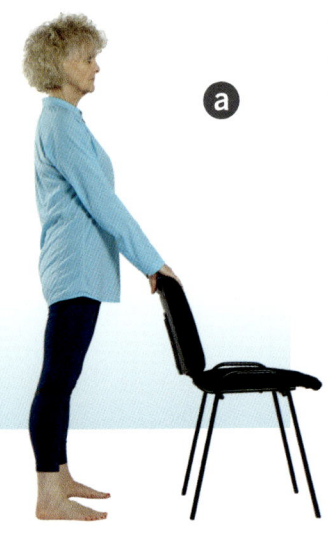

The reason this is such an important exercise for us as we age is that it works so many lower body muscles all at once, which, in turn, makes us stronger and less likely to fall.

Method

- Stand behind your chair and place your hands lightly on the back of it.
- Lengthen through the spine and have your feet placed just a little wider than your hips and either facing forwards or turned out in a ten to two position. **a**
- Breathe in and as you breathe out, bend your knees and stick your bottom out as if you are about to sit down on a chair behind you. Keep your chest open and neck lengthened and focus on something ahead of you. If you have knee or hip issues, just perform a very gentle squat — keep it small and only move within a range that is comfortable for you. **b**
- Take a moment here in the squat position, glance down at your knees and make sure they haven't travelled beyond your toes — you should still be able to see your toes. If you notice that your knees are turning inwards, which can happen, then adjust, gently easing them back so that they are over your ankles. Make sure that you're keeping your heels on the floor.
- Breathe in again while in the squat position and as you breathe out, lift yourself back up to standing.
- Repeat 8 times and increase as you think fit; maybe try squatting lower. Keep at it and you will get stronger. **c**

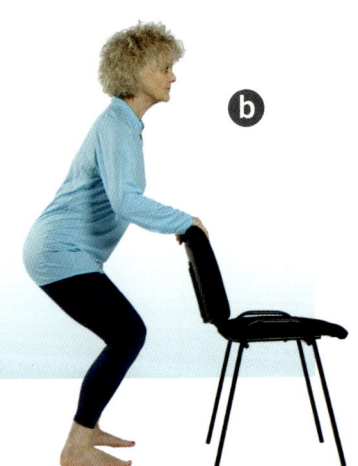

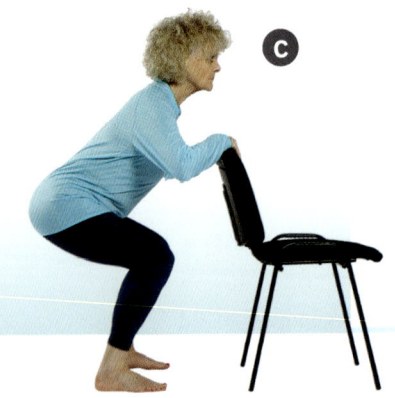

CALF RAISES BALANCE (1)

Method

If you want to make the squat exercise on page 138 more challenging, then while you are in the squat position, rise up on to the ball of your right foot.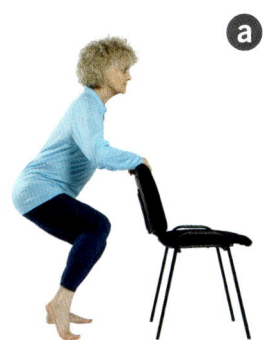

- Hold for a beat and then return your heel to the floor.
- Rise up on to the ball of your left foot.
- Hold for a beat and return your heel to the floor.
- Repeat 4 times, alternating each side.
- Finally, come up on to the balls of both feet at the same time.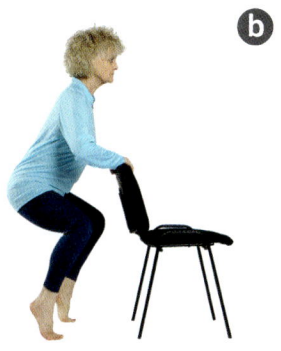
- Hold for a beat, then lower your heels back down to the floor. This is a challenging exercise, so only attempt it if you feel strong enough, as your calves and your quads (thighs) will be working hard. Maybe start with one repetition and see how it feels before continuing.
- Repeat 4 times and then increase repetitions when you feel ready.

STANDING GLUTE EXERCISE (1)

Benefits

This isn't really a balance exercise, but it uses the chair as a prop. This will strengthen those all-important buttock muscles that help you stay upright, walk well and climb stairs. For seated glute exercises see page 93.

Method

- Stand tall behind your chair and hold on to the back of it with both hands.
- Breathe in and as you breathe out, lift your leg and bring your right knee slightly forwards towards your chair.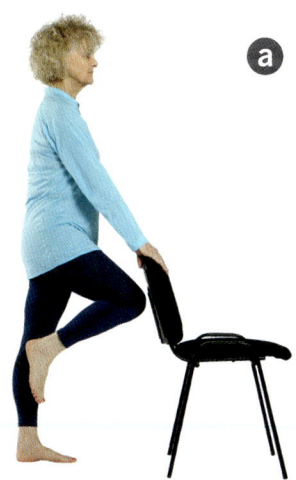

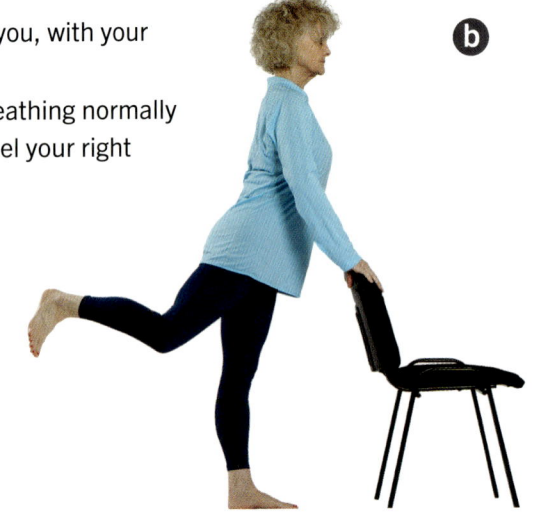

- Gently swing your leg back behind you, with your knee slightly bent.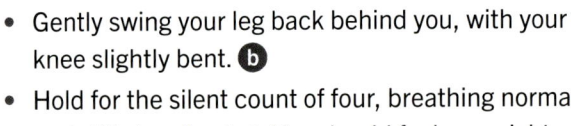
- Hold for the silent count of four, breathing normally and still standing tall. You should feel your right buttock engaging as you hold your leg back behind you.
- Repeat 4 times on each side swinging the leg back and forth.

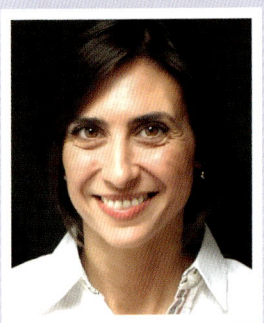

PROFESSIONAL ADVICE

DR HELEN KENNEDY
GENERAL PRACTITIONER

Helen, who has a special interest in women's health, says:

'Exercise is clearly important as we age for both physical and mental benefits. Women need to fight the effects of oestrogen deficiency and maintain muscle strength and bulk as well as flexibility to reduce unwanted symptoms. Weight-bearing exercise is important for bone health, along with an adequate intake of calcium and vitamin D, but for a more holistic approach, consideration should also be given to muscle toning, and Chair Pilates and Yoga is an ideal way to do this. It can be practised at different levels of intensity to suit different abilities and built up at a pace to suit the individual. The benefits of exercise on mental well-being are also well documented. As we get older, and particularly after the menopause, it is normal for us to gain weight, and oestrogen deficiency causes a redistribution of body fat to around the abdomen, giving us more of an apple shape. Exercising can help to maintain a healthy weight and improve posture, both of which can lead to an improvement in body shape and consequently self-confidence. Apart from the satisfaction in knowing that you are being healthy, exercise releases "happy hormones" in the same way that anti-depressant medication can, and is an important part of managing low mood and anxiety, which can also be more common at this time of life.'

CHAPTER 18

RESISTANCE BAND EXERCISES

If you have a resistance band, then you might like to try the following exercises to add variety to your repertoire. There's more information about resistance bands and what sort to purchase if you haven't already got one on page 38. Make sure you've warmed up with a few of the other seated exercises before attempting any of these movements — I suggest some wake-up stretches on page 44, the roll down on page 46, neck stretches on page 51, shoulder rolls on page 54 and spinal rotation on page 59.

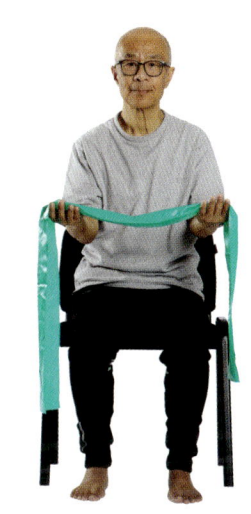

It's up to you how much tension you keep in your band. You'll need to experiment to find out what feels right and suits your ability. As your strength improves you can begin to increase the tension.

Depending on the length and resistance level of your band, you might find that you need to either wrap the band around your hands (if the band is very long) or hold the ends of it in your hands (if the band is shorter).

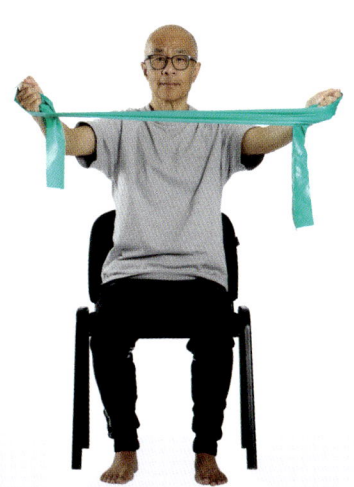

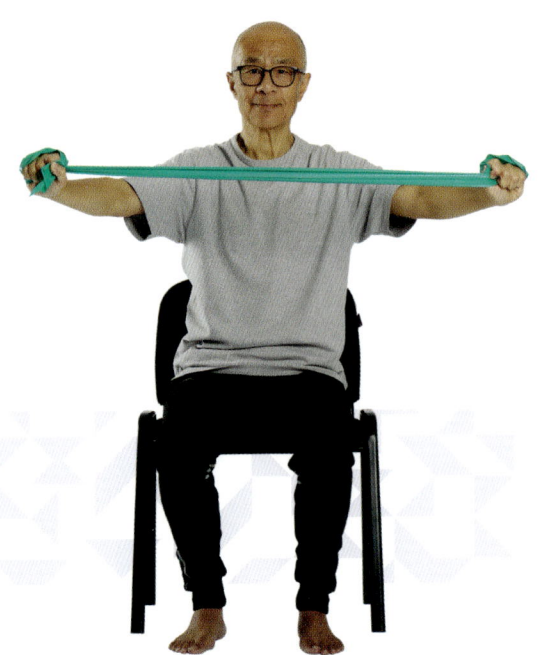

ARMS AND BACK

Benefits

As well as working your arms and strengthening them as you perform the exercise, you'll be working your upper back muscles too – this is great for releasing any tension in your back, especially if you've been sitting at a computer all day.

Method

- Sit up tall but slightly forwards, towards the front of your chair so that you aren't tempted to lean back or slouch, with your feet on the floor beneath your knees.
- Wrap your resistance band around your hands and extend your arms straight out in front of your torso.
- Try to keep your wrists in a neutral position and avoid bending them up or down. You might need to adjust your grip a bit so that you have the right amount of resistance in your band; you'll know when that is, as you'll feel the muscles in your arms activate.
- Take a breath in and as you breathe out, gently pull the ends of the band, opening your arms and easing the band outwards so that your arms move a small distance to the side.
- Hold as you breathe in, and then as you breathe out, release back to the start position.
- Repeat up to 8 times.

SHOULDERS

Benefits

This exercise targets the rotator cuff muscles, which are a group of muscles in your shoulder that allow for a wide range of movement and keep your shoulder joint stabilised. If you suffer from a frozen shoulder or arthritis in this area, you might find that this exercise is recommended by your health professional, but if you do have problems, please use a light resistance band to start with. You'll find the same exercise without a resistance band on page 72.

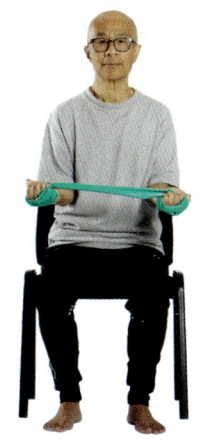

Method

- Sit up tall on your chair.
- Wrap the band around your hands, bend your elbows to 90 degrees and glue them to your ribcage, keeping your forearms and hands facing upwards. **a**
- Breathe in and as you breathe out, gently ease the band out to the sides keeping your elbows glued to your ribcage. It probably won't go far; it's a small but effective movement. **b**
- Hold as you breathe in again, and then as you breathe out, release the tension in the band.
- Repeat 4 times.

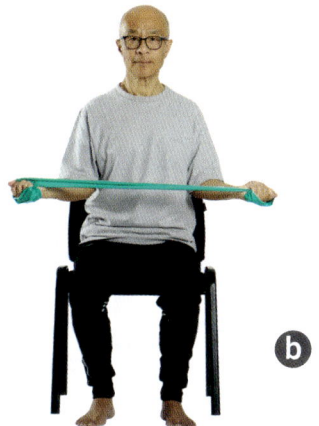

- Now pull on one side of the band, then the other, still keeping your elbows glued to your ribcage and lengthening through your spine. **c**
- Repeat 4 times on each side, alternating right and left side.

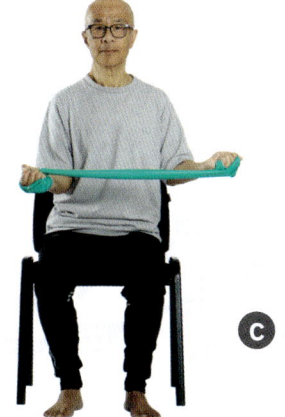

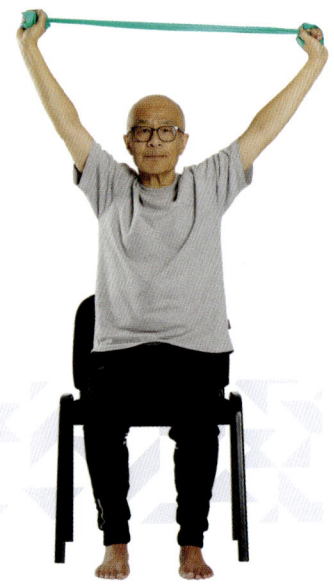

SIDE BEND WITH ARMS

Benefits

This exercise will help strengthen and stretch the muscles in your arms, but also provide your torso with a wonderful side stretch, as well as working your abdominal muscles.

Method

- Sit up tall on your chair.
- Wrap the band around your hands or hold the ends.
- Breathe in and as you breathe out, raise your arms above your head, placing them slightly wider than your shoulders (you may need to adjust the band to suit). Keep your arms straight.
- Breathe in as you hold and then as you breathe out, lean to your right, keeping the band taut between your hands.
- Breathe in again as you hold the stretch to the right for a moment.
- As you breathe out, shift your arms back to centre and move them over to the left. Keep those abdominal muscles engaged.
- Hold the stretch to the left as you breathe in, and as you breathe out, return to centre.
- Repeat 4 times.
- Roll your shoulders after this exercise to release any tension that may have built up.

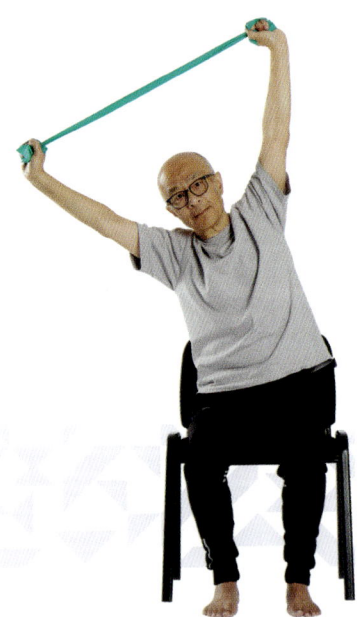

BICEP CURL

Biceps are the muscles at the front of your upper arm. They help bend the elbow and supinate (rotate with your palm upwards) the arm.

Benefits

We use our bicep muscles for everything — from lifting up a mug of tea or coffee to turning a doorknob, picking things up or pulling something towards us. But like the rest of the body, we need to work on them to keep them functioning efficiently as we age and to maintain muscle mass. See pages 70—1 for a bicep exercise without the resistance band.

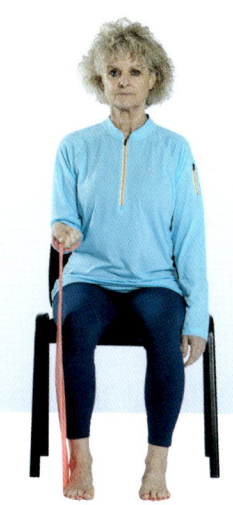

Method

- Place the end of your band under your right foot, making sure that it is secure.
- Wrap the band around your right hand or hold the end of your band.
- Bend your elbow to a 90-degree angle with your palms facing upwards keeping the band taut.
- Breathe in and as you breathe out, raise your forearm, gently pulling the band upwards, so that your hand reaches your shoulder.
- Hold the position as you breathe in, and then as you breathe out, lower your arm back down to the 90-degree start position.
- Adjust the band if it's too strong or too light.
- Repeat 4 times.

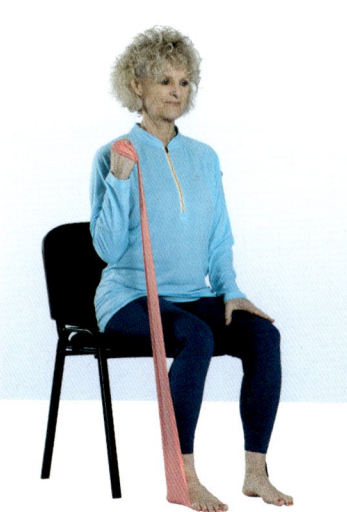

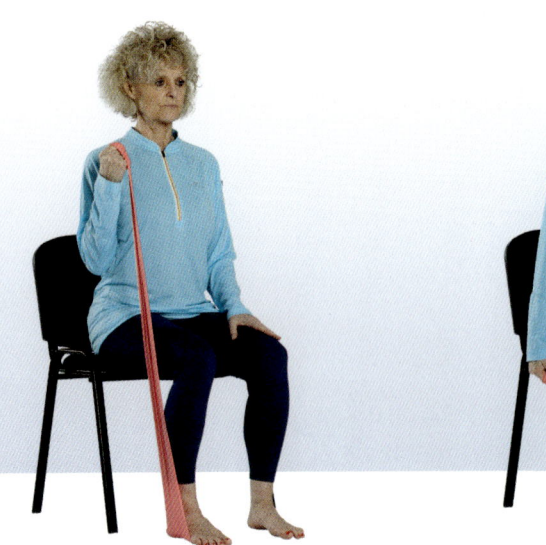
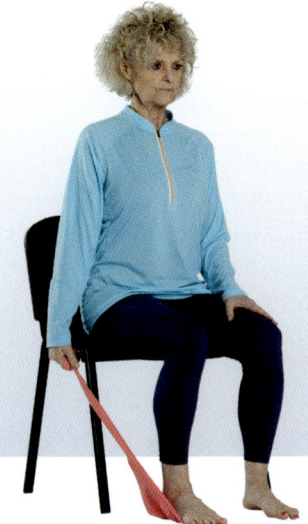

- Take your forearm all the way down to the side of your body.
- Breathe in and as you breathe out, lift it all the way back up to your shoulders. Try to keep your shoulders relaxed as you do so.
- Breathe in again and then as you breathe out, lower your arm back down to your side.
- Repeat 4 times.
- Repeat everything on the other side.

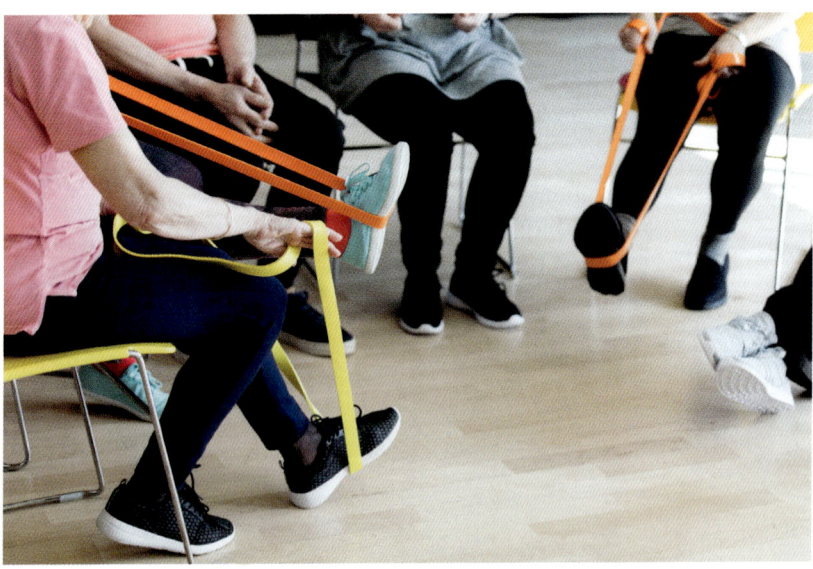

FOREARMS

Benefits

The forearm muscles (the muscles of your lower arms) are important for grip strength — holding the handle of a coffee mug, opening the top of a jar or turning a doorknob, for example. They also help move your elbow, wrist and fingers.

Method

- Place the end of the resistance band underneath the sole of your right foot, making sure that it is secure.
- Wrap the other end of the band around your hand or hold on to the end of the band with your palms facing downwards.
- Bend your elbows to a 90-degree angle.
- Breathe in and as you breathe out, lift your forearm upwards. It might not be able to go far and that's fine.
- Breathe in again and as you breathe out, return to the start position.
- Repeat 4 times and then swap to the other arm.

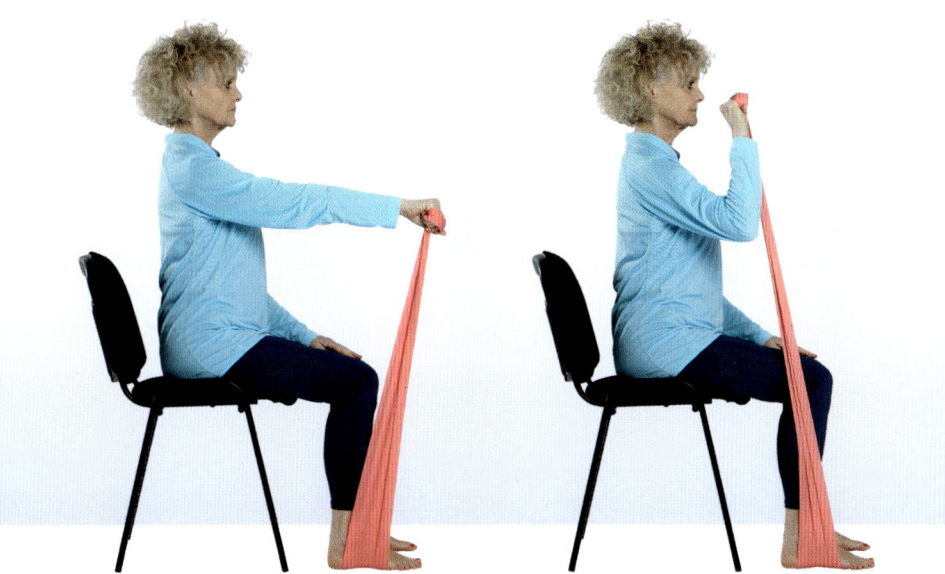

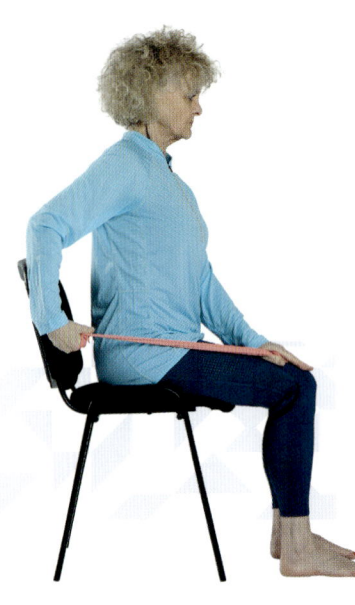

TRICEPS

Benefits

The tricep muscles sit on the underside of your arms and play an important role in moving your arms away from your body, moving your arms back behind your body, and carrying things overhead.

There are two tricep exercises using resistance bands for you to try here. See page 73 for an exercise without the resistance band.

TRICEPS 1

Method

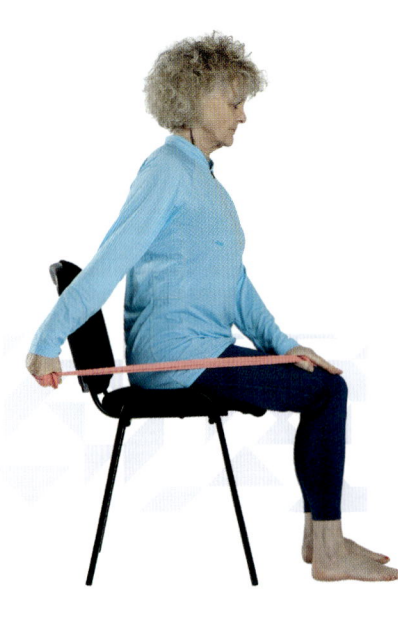

- Sit forwards on your chair for this exercise, as you need space to be able to manoeuvre your arm behind you.
- Place the end of the resistance band on your right thigh and place your left hand on top of it to hold it down and keep it in place.
- Wrap the other end of the band around your right hand or hold on to the end of the band.
- Bend your right elbow and move it backwards as if nudging someone out of the way.
- Keeping your elbow in the backward position, extend your arm.
- Hold for a beat and then release back to the bent elbow position.
- Repeat 8 times and then change sides.

TRICEPS 2

This exercise will challenge your coordination just with the set-up! But follow the pictures and my words and it will become second nature, so that you can reap the benefits of this tricep exercise.

Method

- Sit up tall on your chair.
- Hold the end of your band in your left hand and then bend your elbow and take your arm around to your back.
- Take hold of the other end of your band with your right hand and keep the band about shoulder height and directly above your left hand.
- Make sure there is some resistance in your band — you might need to wrap the end of it around your right hand to pull it taut.
- Breathe in and as you breathe out, extend your right arm above your head, pulling the band tight and engaging your tricep muscles.
- Breathe in again and hold for a beat and then as you breathe out, bend your right elbow back to the start position.
- Repeat 8 times and then change sides.

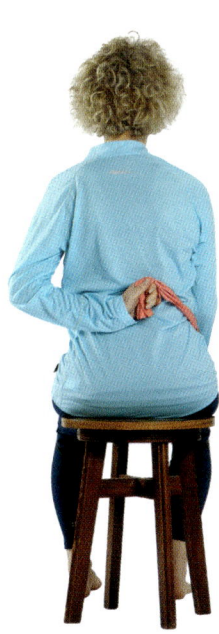
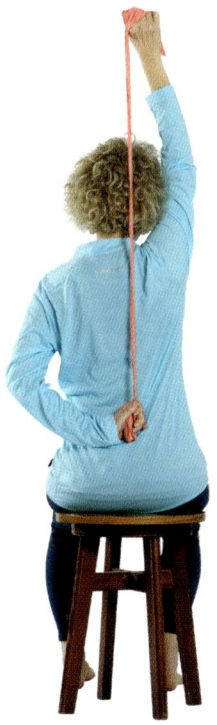

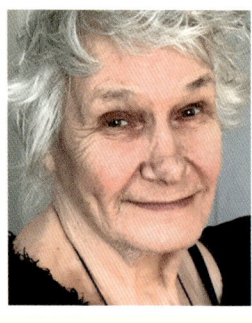

CASE STUDY

ANN MURKETT
AGE 81

'I used to swim, run and be very active and then I had a couple of falls that damaged the left side of my body. I've also had spondylitis of the spine for 40-odd years. The brain is still okay, I do Sudoku and play solitaire, I think that's important. I have to try and be active as best I can by gardening, pottering and getting out once a week, and I cycle my legs while lying on my back in bed every morning, but the Chair Pilates and Yoga really helps me to keep at it and strengthen my weak arm and leg.'

SHOULDERS/DELTOIDS

These muscles, which sit on the outside of your upper arm, connect the upper arm to the body.

Benefits

These muscles help move your arms in all directions, enabling you to push, pull and lift. They also protect and stabilise your shoulder joint, so that if you're carrying bags of shopping with your arms down by your sides, for example, you don't injure your shoulder. For a deltoid exercise without the resistance band see page 74.

Method

- Place your feet on top of the centre of the band.
- Sit up tall, lengthen through your spine.
- Wrap each hand around the band or hold on to the ends securely and bend your arms slightly with your hands facing downwards.

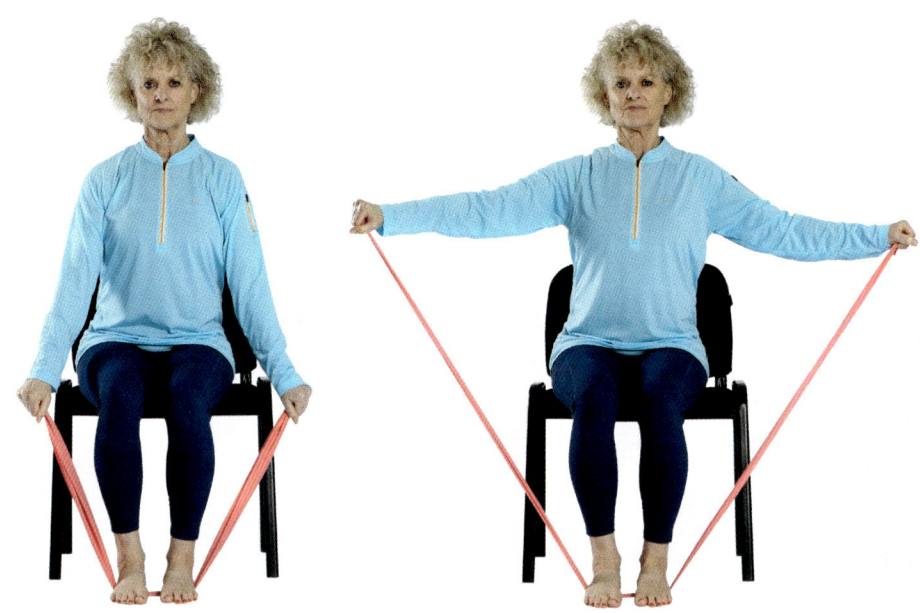

- Breathe in and as you breathe out, raise your arms and pull the band up to the side, aiming for shoulder height if you can.
- Breathe in as you hold the position and breathe out as you release the band and return to the start position.
- Adjust the band if it's too loose or too tight.
- Repeat 4 times to begin with and then progress to more repetitions when you feel ready.
- If you find performing this exercise with both arms at the same time challenging, alternate the arms, lifting one side at a time, or do 4 on one side and then 4 on the other.

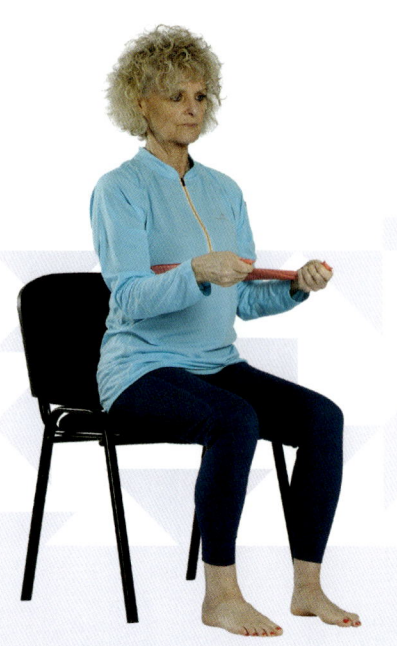
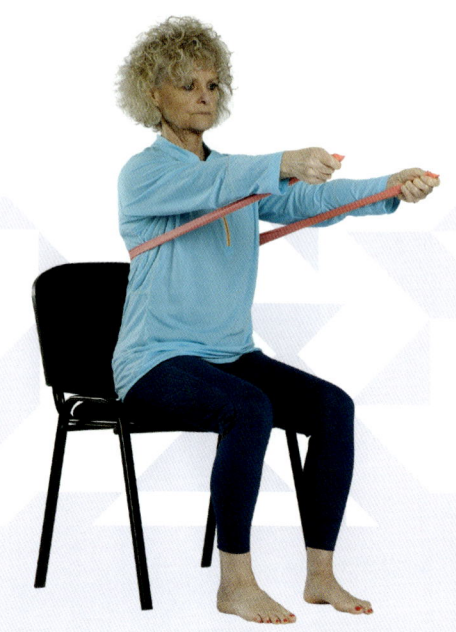

CHEST PRESS

Benefits

This is an exercise for strengthening the chest and arms.

Method

- Sit up tall and wrap the band around your mid—upper back.
- Wrap the band around your hands or hold the ends and bend your elbows to the side of your body. The tension in the band will be loose at this point.
- Breathe in and as you breathe out, gently pull the band forwards, extending your arms out in front of your chest. Make sure you have adequate tension in the band.
- Breathe in again as you pause in this position and then breathe out slowly, releasing the tension in your band.
- Repeat 8 times.
- If you prefer, you can alternate the arms, extending one at a time.

LOWER BODY

Benefits

All these exercises will help strengthen the legs, knees and bottom muscles. They will also improve coordination and flexibility and might make you sweat!

Method

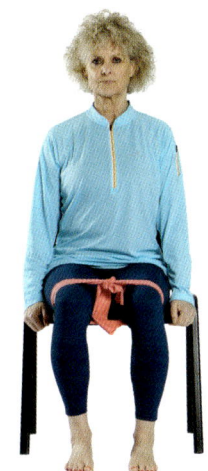

For these resistance band exercises you will need to tie the band around your thighs. Make sure you tie it securely so that it doesn't suddenly ping off your legs when you perform the movement! If you own a small round resistance band you can use this instead.

- Shift yourself slightly forwards on your chair, and lengthen through your spine. **a**
- Breathe in and as you breathe out push your knees against the band. **b**
- Hold as you breathe in again and then release on your out-breath. You might like to try and engage your buttock muscles as well like you did for the Butt Clench exercise on page 93.
- Repeat 8 times.
- Now lift your heels off the floor so that you are on the balls of your feet. **c**
- Breathing normally for this exercise, pulse your knees outwards against the resistance band in small, fast movements for the count of eight.
- Relax and repeat.

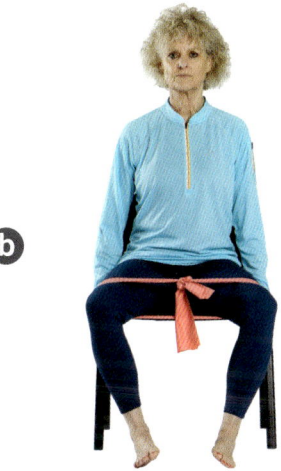

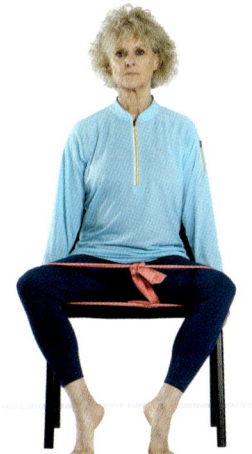

LEG PRESS

Method

- Sit up tall on your chair, lengthen through the spine.
- Extend your right leg out in front of your chair, hooking the middle of the band around the sole of your foot.
- Wrap the band around your hands or hold the ends securely. Make sure that there is tension in the band.
- Breathe in and as you breathe out, bend your knee and bring it towards your torso. Your arms will move backwards as you do so.
- Breathe in again and as you breathe out, extend your leg, pushing against the resistance band.
- Repeat 8 times and then swap sides.

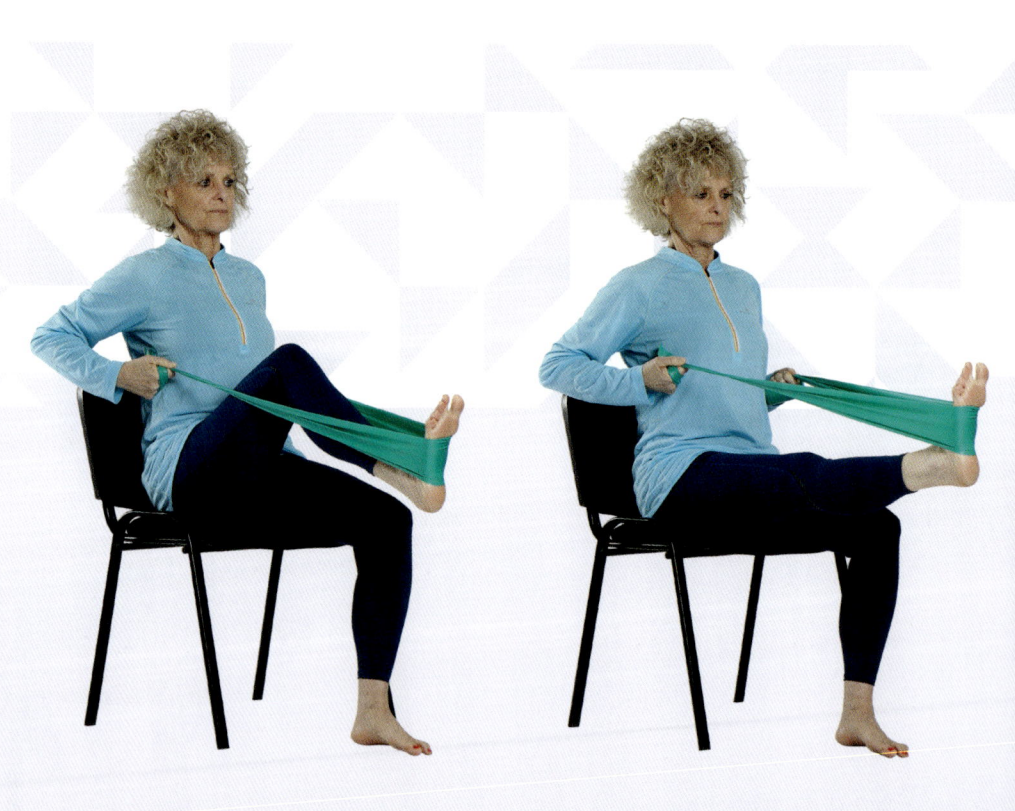

FEET AND ANKLES

For feet exercises without the resistance band see page 114. If your feet are feeling particularly stiff, please make sure you have completed some of the exercises in chapter 14 before attempting this one.

Benefits

Not only will this exercise improve your foot and ankle strength, but also your calf muscles (lower leg) will get a workout.

Method

- Sit up tall on your chair.
- Extend your right leg out in front of your chair, hooking the middle of the band around the sole of your foot.
- Wrap the band around your hands or hold the ends securely. Make sure there is tension in the band.
- Breathe normally and with your right leg extended, point your toes, pushing against the resistance of the band.
- Then flex (turn your toes upwards), still keeping the tension in the band so that the sole of your foot has to work against the pull of the band.
- Continue to point and flex the foot 8 times. Repeat on the other side.

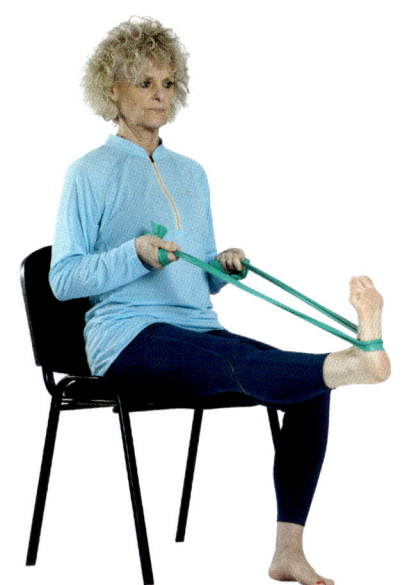

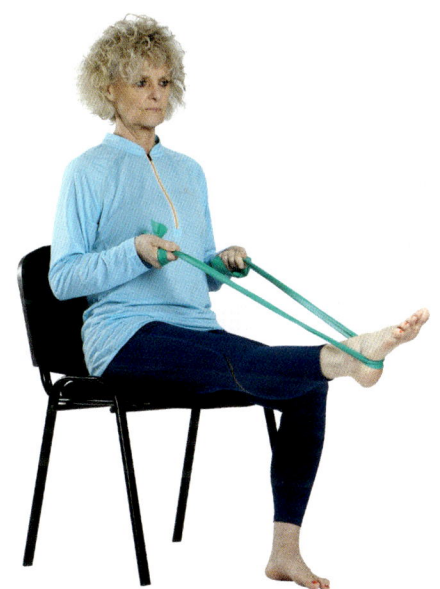

CHAPTER 19

CARDIO EXERCISES

The following seated exercises are more dynamic, with the aim of increasing your heart rate. Only attempt these if you feel comfortable to do so and if in doubt, please talk with a health professional to make sure that they are suitable for you. None of these exercises are hard to do, but the dynamic, slightly faster nature of the movements will work your body and cardiovascular system more. You might like to put some funky music on for this section and perform the exercises to the beat!

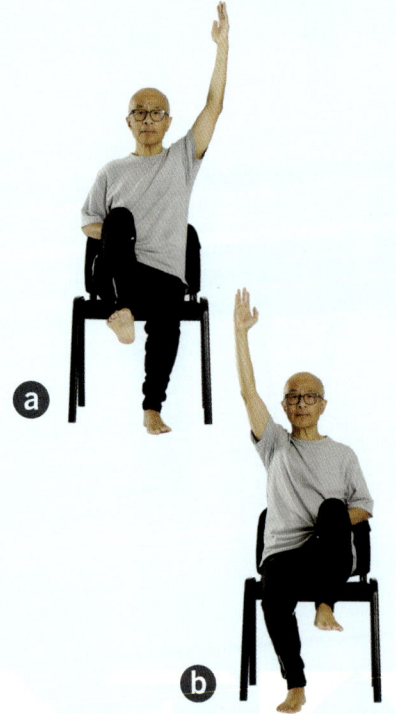

If you'd like to make these exercises more challenging, use light hand and/or ankle weights.

Make sure you are warmed up before trying this exercise routine – perform the roll down on page 46, and some neck (page 50), shoulder (page 54), basic leg lift (page 99) and gentle arm (page 70) exercises.

- Sit up tall, lengthen through your spine with your feet on the floor hip-width apart.
- Raise your left arm and your right leg. **a**
- Raise your right arm and left leg. **b**
- Complete 20 repetitions at a speed that suits.
- Rest and repeat.

- Raise your left arm in the air and kick your right leg out in front of your chair. 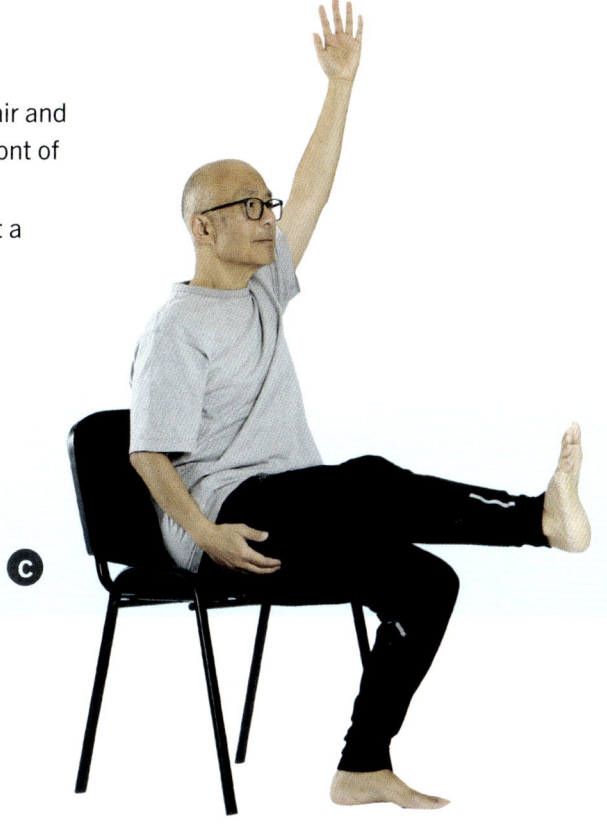 **c**
- Complete 20 repetitions at a speed that suits.
- Repeat on the other side.
- Rest and repeat.

c

Only your legs this time:

- Bend your right knee, lengthen your leg, bend your knee again and place your foot back down on the floor.
- Alternate the legs for 20 repetitions at a speed that suits.
- Rest and then repeat.

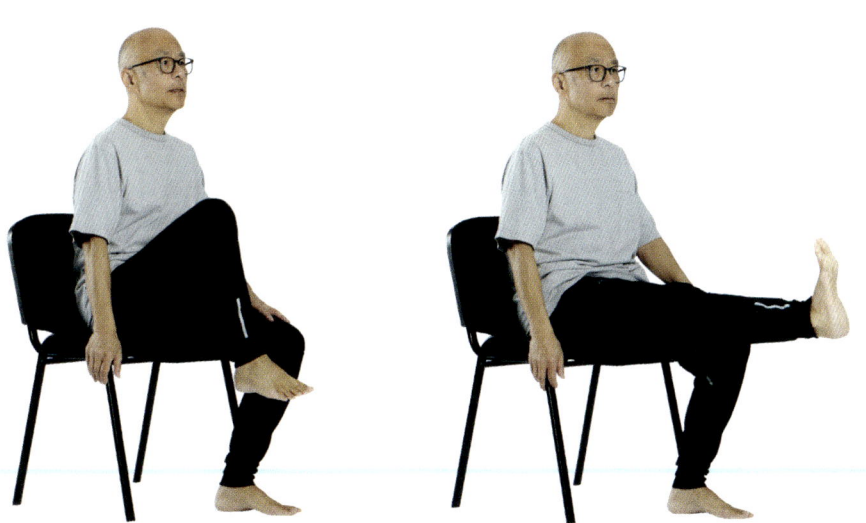

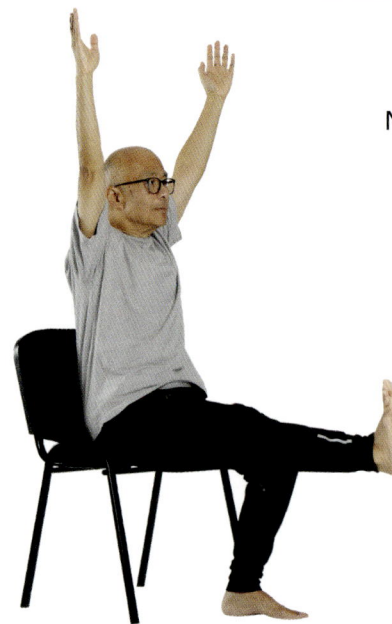

Now we're going to use the arms again:

- Sit up tall on your chair.
- Lengthen both arms above your head.
- As you lower your arms down to your sides, lift your right leg.
- Place your right foot down on the floor and raise your arms in the air above your head again.
- Repeat on the other side and alternate for 20 repetitions at a speed that suits.

This time we are adding in some stretching too:

- Sit up tall on your chair.
- Extend your right leg out in front of your chair.
- Raise your left arm and reach over towards your foot, aiming to get as close to your foot as possible – or aim to touch your thigh or knee.
- Raise your arm up again.
- Repeat 10 times, keeping your leg extended throughout.
- Repeat on the other side.

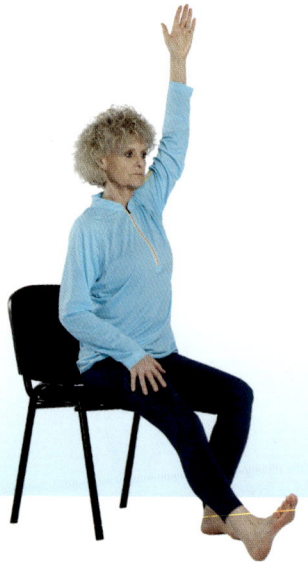

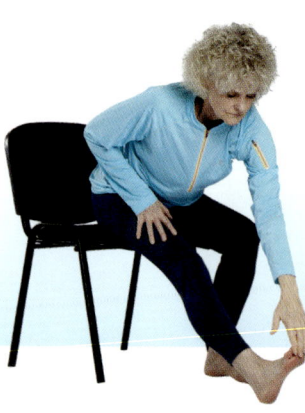

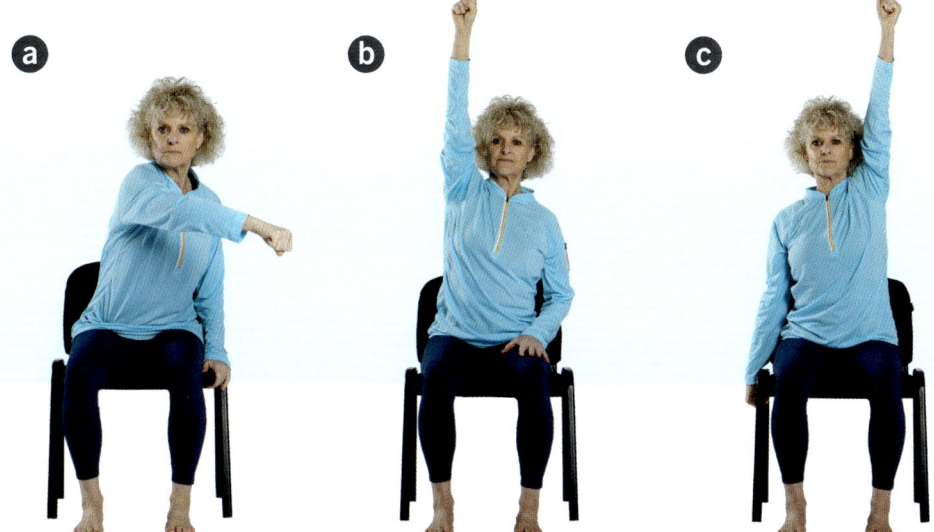

Similar to Pack a Punch 1 and 2 on pages 84 and 85, you're now going to perform some dynamic punches.

- Make sure you're still sitting tall, lengthen through your spine with your feet on the floor below your knees
- Punch across your body, alternating your arms, for 20 repetitions. (a)
- Then punch in the air above your head for 20 repetitions. (b) (c)

CASE STUDY

SIMON LESLIE
AGE 50

'I had a brain tumour in 2019 and had to learn to walk again. These chair exercises have really helped me regain my mobility – it took two months for me to be able to walk again, but now I try and walk every single day and the seated exercises, especially the sit-to-stand one not using my hands to ease myself up, are helping me get stronger.'

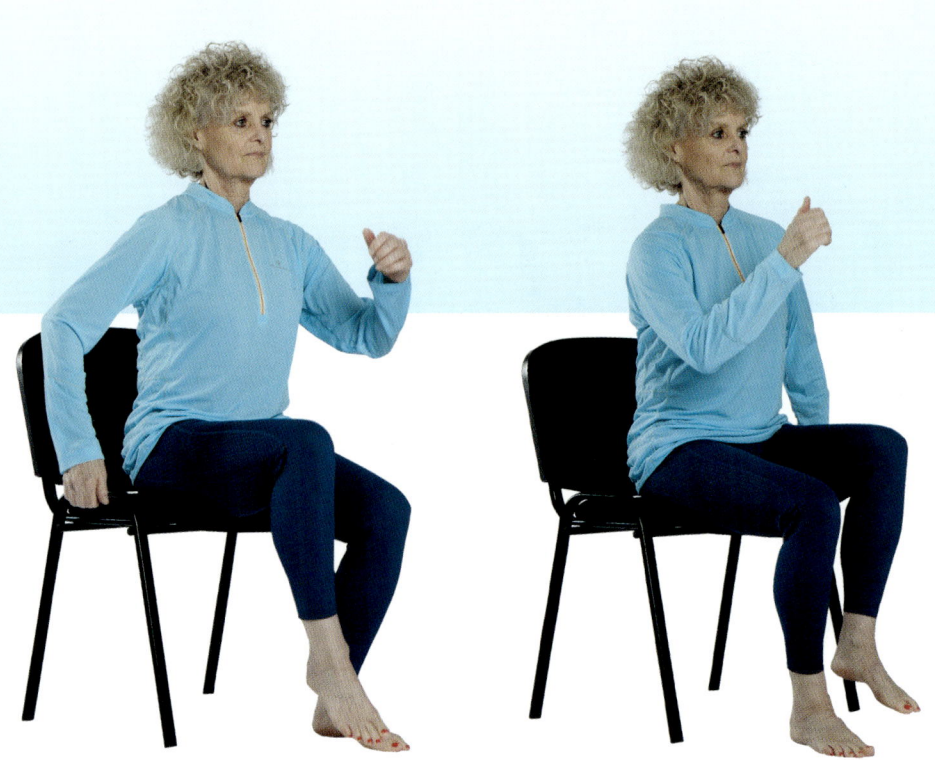

Now we're going to try some seated running!

- Sit up tall and engage your abdominal muscles.
- Breathe normally and begin to pretend run on the spot alternating your feet and arms at a speed that suits.
- Aim for 30 repetitions.
- Rest and repeat.

Finally, we're going to repeat the sit-to-stand exercise on page 128. But this time faster and with your arms in the air as you raise yourself off the chair.

- Sit up tall on your chair.
- Breathing normally, engage your abdominal muscles and/or pelvic floor muscles.
- Stand up, raising your arms above your head as you do so.
- Repeat 10 times at a speed that suits.
- Rest and repeat.

Follow the cardio session with some relaxing stretches that you'll find in the next chapter.

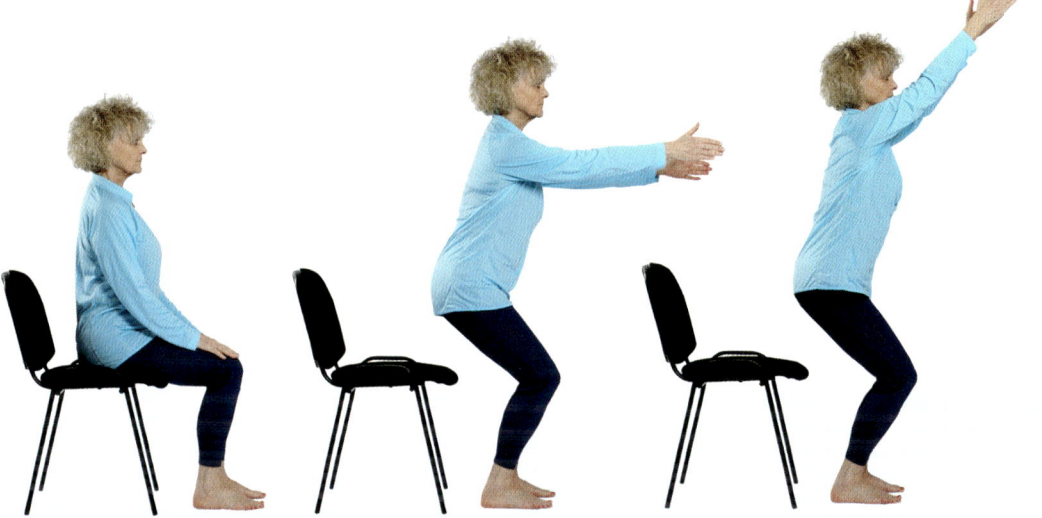

CHAPTER 20

STRETCHES

Once you have completed some of the exercises in this book, you might like to focus more on stretching. Having said that, many of the Chair Pilates and Yoga movements include flexibility. However, sometimes all you might feel like doing is stretching. It's a good idea to stretch after the more strenuous exercises, so it will depend on how you feel after you have finished your routine.

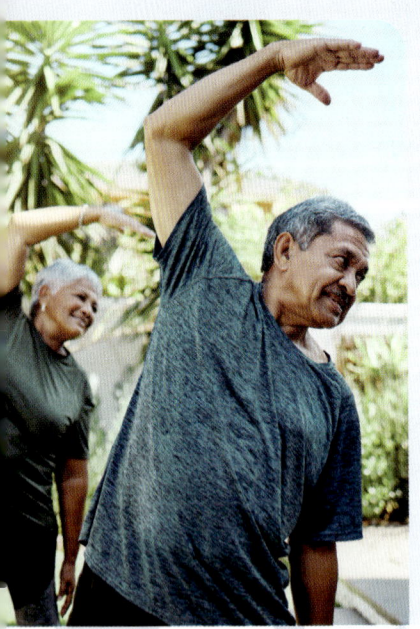

BACK STRETCHES (B)

For the first of these exercises, a seated back stretch, you'll need two chairs, and ideally, the chair in front of where you sit needs to be able to slide a little distance away from you. However, if the chair that you're sitting on is placed on the carpet, then this probably won't be possible. The exercise can still work; it just won't be quite as satisfying as a full back stretch.

Benefits

This exercise not only lengthens the muscles in your mid- and upper back, which can get stiff and tight if you tend to be sedentary, but also strengthens it.

Method

- Place your other chair in front of you so that it faces you.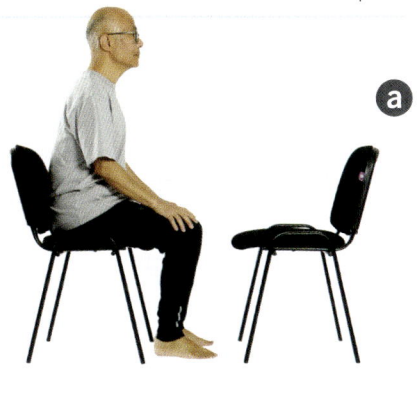

- Breathe in and as you breathe out, hinge your torso over towards the chair seat in front of you and place your forearms on its seat.

- Keep your head in line with your spine, and try not to tilt your head up or down.

- With your forearms still on the seat in front of you, breathe in again and as you breathe out, lift your torso up, keeping your forearms on the chair (like the sphinx pose in yoga or the swan dive on forearms in mat Pilates) and your neck in line with your spine.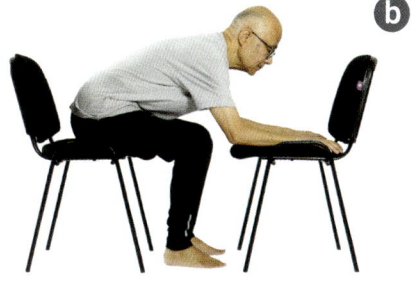

- Breathe out and lower yourself back down to the start position.

- Repeat 4 times.

- Now clasp the edge of the chair in front of you with both hands.

- Breathe in and as you breathe out, gently push the chair away from you: not far, just so that your arms become outstretched. Keep looking down at the floor, with your neck and spine aligned.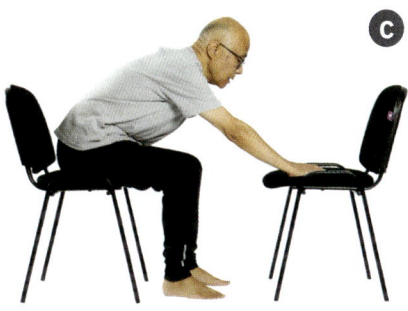

- Hold this stretch, breathing normally, for a silent count of 10.

- Breathe in and as you breathe out, gently pull the chair back to the start position.

- Then repeat.

Note: If your chair doesn't move because it is placed on carpet or it isn't a very moveable chair, just lengthen your forearms as far forwards as they will go. If you have a backless chair, you can slide your hands through the back of it. But if not, just move to wherever the chair size allows.

UPPER BACK STRETCH (B)

Benefits

This movement can alleviate any tension from a tight upper back (thoracic spine) and chest muscles. If you find yourself bent over a computer all day, or tend to slouch, this movement can help stretch out those tight muscles and improve posture.

Method

- Sit up tall on your chair.
- Take both your hands behind the back of your head, elbows out to the side, and make sure you are sitting as far back on the chair as you can so that your back is supported.
- Breathe in and as you breathe out, lean back as far as it's comfortable to do so, looking up at the ceiling; you should feel your chest muscles open and your upper back extend over the back of your chair.
- Hold for a silent count of 10, breathing normally.
- Breathe in and as you breathe out, lift up and return to the start position.
- Repeat 4 times. Increase the repetitions if you feel the need.

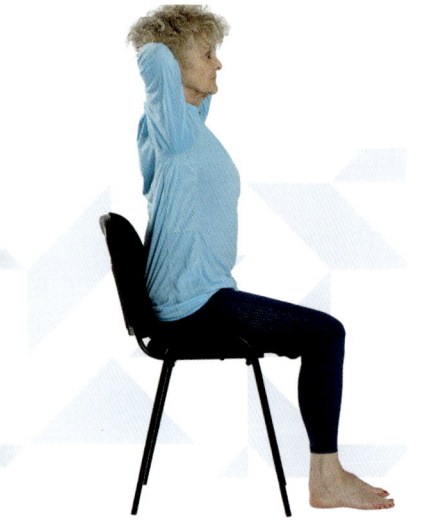

BACK, ARM AND LEG STRETCHES USING THE CHAIR AS A PROP (B)

Benefits

This satisfying stretch will allow your back to stretch itself out and lengthen your legs, particularly your hamstrings (back of thighs), which can become very tight if you sit a lot. It will also stretch your arms.

This time you are going to use your chair as a prop like you did for the balance exercises in chapter 17.

Method

- Stand behind your chair holding on to the back of it.
- Take a step or two backwards and place your feet hip-width apart.
- Breathe in and as you breathe out, drop your torso forwards and shift your hips backwards, still holding on to the chair. Your feet should face forwards.
- Drop your chest and straighten your arms a little. Try not to hold on to the back of the chair for dear life: it should be a light touch.
- Hold this stretch for a silent count of 10, breathing normally. Feel the stretch travel up the back of your legs, into your buttocks, back muscles and arms. Keep your neck in line with your spine.
- Breathe in again and lift up.
- As you breathe out, return to the full stretch position.
- Repeat 4 times.

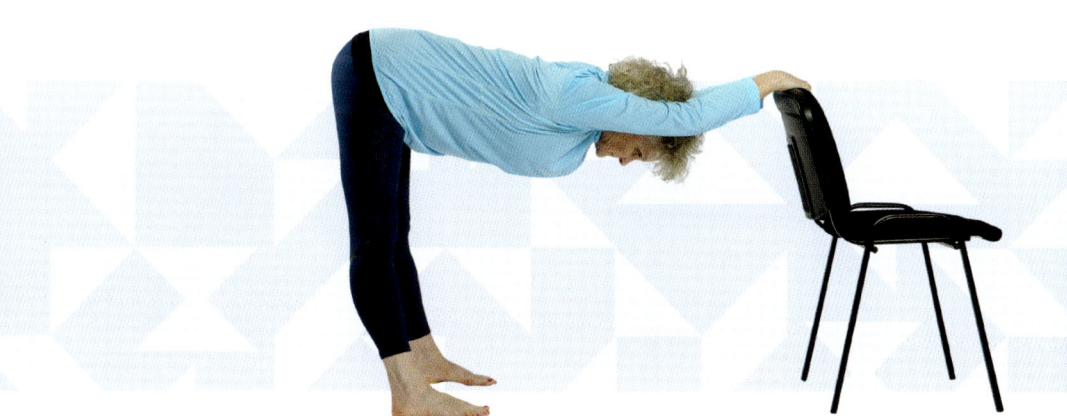

TRIANGLE (1)

Benefits

In a traditional yoga class, the triangle pose would be performed standing up. This seated version will stretch your torso and open out your chest to allow deeper breathing. It is a wonderful energising stretch.

Method

- Sit up tall and take your legs out to either side of your chair.
- Breathe in and as you breathe out, raise your arms to shoulder height in aeroplane mode.
- Breathe in and as you breathe out, gently twist to your left and place your right hand on your ankle, shin or knee and your left arm up in the air above.
- Hold for the count of two enjoying the stretch. Turn your head up towards your raised hand if it's comfortable to do so. If not, look down at the floor – whatever is comfortable for your neck.
- Breathe in and as you breathe out, return to an upright position.
- Repeat on the other side.
- Repeat 4 times, holding the stretch for a couple of breaths on each side.

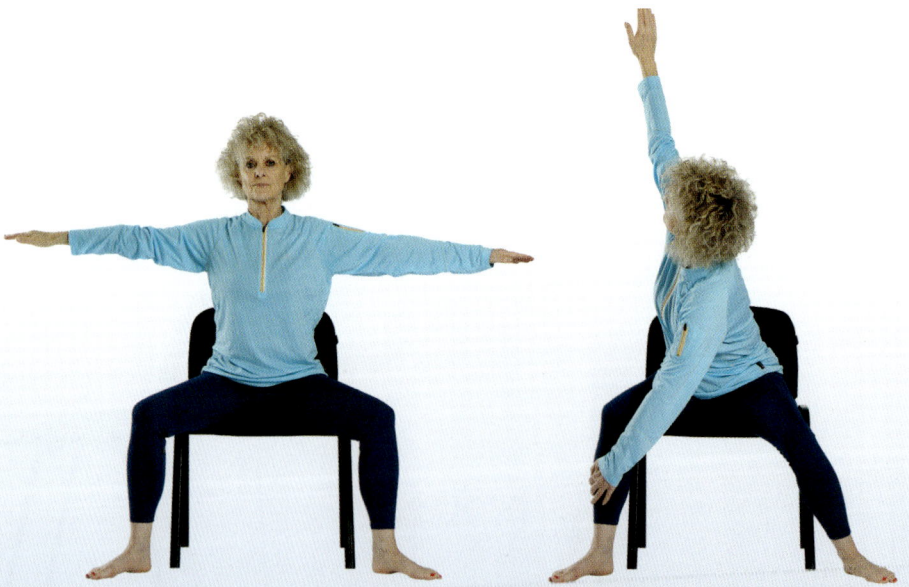

BICEPS ARM STRETCH (B)

Benefits

This simple arm stretch will help lengthen the muscles of your upper arm, specifically the bicep muscles, and is great to do after you've exercised your arms on page 70 or completed the resistance band workout on page 145.

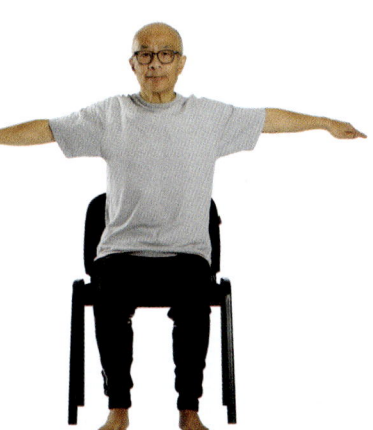

Method

- Sit up tall on your chair..
- Breathe in and as you breathe out, raise your arms to shoulder height and into the aeroplane wing position with your palms facing upwards and your shoulders relaxed.
- Keeping this position, take your arms a little further behind your body until you feel a stretch in your upper arm — you'll know when you reach it.
- Hold for a slow, silent count of 10.
- Rest your arms.
- Repeat, taking the arms to the side again, but this time turn your palms downwards until your thumb is pointing towards the floor.
- Hold for a slow, silent count of 10. Remember to breathe and try not to let your back arch.
- Rest your arms.

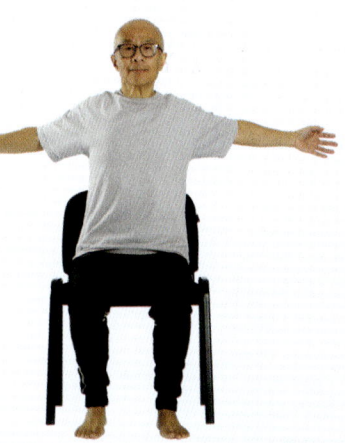

- Move further forwards on your chair now and depending on your shoulder mobility, take your arms behind your back, clasping your hands together if comfortable. This will draw your shoulder blades together.
- Gently lift your hands a little way upwards until you feel the stretch.
- Hold for a couple of breaths and then release.

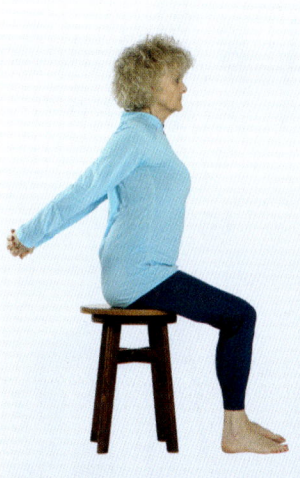

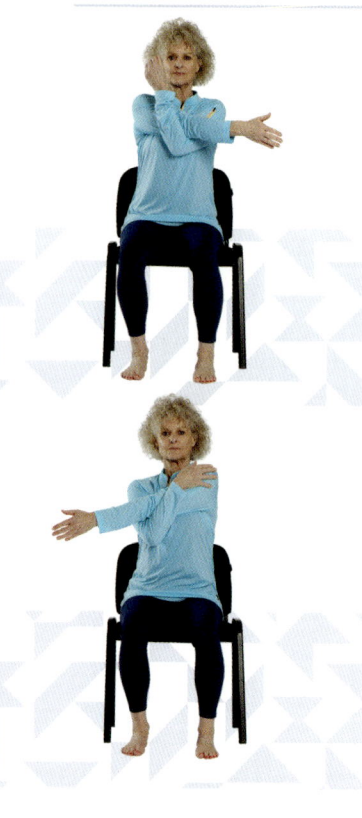

TRICEPS ARM STRETCH (B)

Benefits

This will lengthen the muscles of the underarm: the 'bat wings' that might be feeling a bit tight after some of the arm exercises on pages 70–7 or the resistance band exercises in chapter 18.

Method

- Sit up tall on your chair.
- Take one arm horizontally over your torso towards the other side of your body.
- Keep it straight and wrap your other arm, bending the elbow, around the top part of the extended arm.
- Gently ease the arm a little further over until you feel the stretch.
- Hold for a silent count of 10, then release.
- Repeat on the other side.

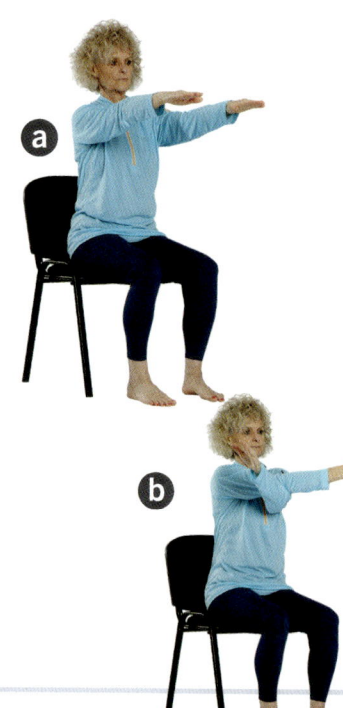

EAGLE ARMS STRETCH (I)

Benefits

This yoga posture is a strong stretch for the shoulders and upper back and can be quite challenging.

Method

- Sit up tall on your chair.
- Extend both your arms in front of your body. **a**
- Breathe in and as you breathe out, cross your right elbow over your left elbow. **b**

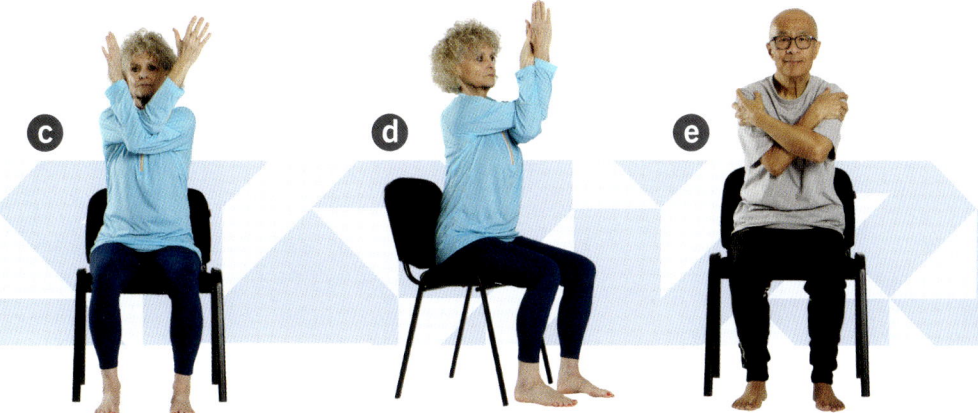

- Bring the back of your forearms together. 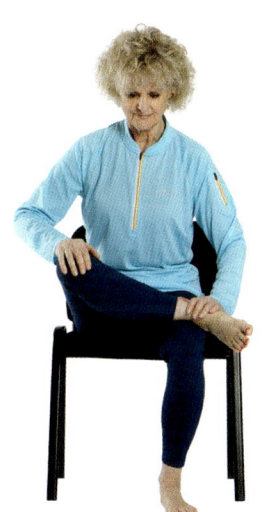 ⓒ
- Bring the palms of your hands together.
- Holding your hands together, raise your elbows up to shoulder height. ⓓ
- Breathe normally and hold the stretch for a count of four before releasing the arms.
- Perform the stretch on the other side.
- If this is too challenging, and for many it is, just hug your body — wrap your arms around your torso and give yourself a big hug. ⓔ

PIRIFORMIS STRETCH (1)

Benefits

The piriformis is in your buttock and can sometimes cause irritation relating to sciatica. This exercise can provide relief, but if you've had any hip or knee surgery or have problems in either area, please omit this stretch.

Method

- Sit up tall and lengthen through the spine.
- Raise your right knee and cross your right ankle over your left thigh into a figure 4 position.
- Lean slightly forwards, towards your leg.
- Hold this stretch for a silent count of 10 and then repeat on the other side.

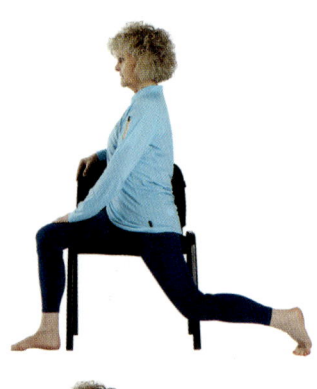

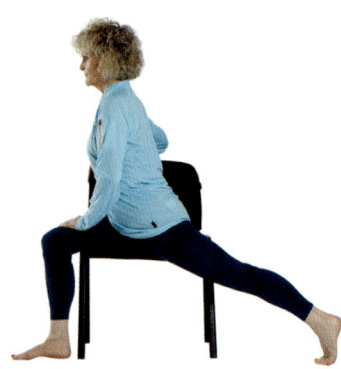

HIP FLEXOR (I)

Benefits

Hip flexors help lift your legs as you walk but can become very tight if you sit for long periods, so this stretch will alleviate some of that tightness.

Method

- Turn sideways on your chair and hold on to the back of it.
- Take your outside leg back behind you as if you're about to kneel (careful of knees).
- Lengthen the leg further out behind you or if that is too strong a stretch, just hold the first position with your knee still bent.
- Lean your torso towards the back of the chair.
- Hold for the silent count of 10 and then repeat on the other side.

SPINAL STRETCH (B)

Benefits

This is a very satisfying stretch for the back muscles. You'll also feel a stretch in your legs.

Method

- Sit up tall and lengthen your legs out in front of you.
- Flex your feet (toes pointing upwards).
- Breathe in and as you breathe out, lengthen your arms with the aim of touching your toes. If you can't touch your toes, aim for your shins or knees.
- Hold for a silent count of 10.
- Breathe in again and as you breathe out, raise your torso back up to the sitting position.
- Repeat 4 times.

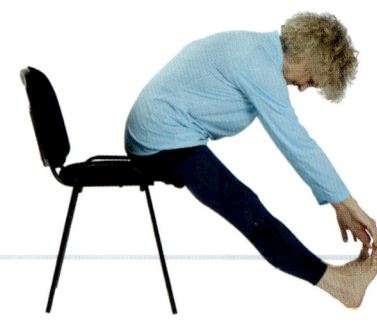

CHAPTER 21

SLEEP AND RELAXATION

As we age our sleeping habits can change. It is estimated that between 40 and 70 per cent of older adults sleep badly. Sleep deprivation can contribute to many health issues in our later life because if we don't get enough sleep, our bodies and minds don't have a chance to recharge their batteries.

Sleep problems can be another reason for falls or other injuries. If you're tired all the time then your concentration tends not to be good, your mind can become sluggish and you can begin to feel depressed. In fact, a decreased mental capacity is a common trait of insomnia. There are, of course, many reasons for bad or restless sleep (overstimulation, medication, frequent visits to the loo, illness, restless legs…), but using your body and performing the exercises in this book will help your muscles to relax and rest at night, and this can go some way towards improving the situation and might even cure it.

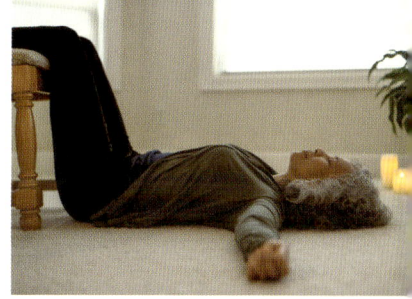

Time spent relaxing and slowing down just before bedtime can also help. Both restorative yoga and yoga nidra are well known for their relaxing and de-stressing qualities and both are well worth exploring. Here you'll find a couple of examples of them, a restorative pose using the chair or pillows as a prop (restorative yoga will mostly require you to stay down on the floor, but there is very little getting up and down and you rest in a pose for many minutes, so it's suitable for those with mobility issues).

Yoga nidra, which means 'yoga sleep' in Sanskrit, is a wonderful way to relax your body and fall into a pre-sleep state. It's also a way to get in touch with how your body feels and learn to let go. This is something many of us struggle with and another reason we can end up not sleeping as our minds chitter-chatter away to us endlessly into the night trying to solve this or that problem.

Yoga nidra is best practised by listening to someone taking you through the relaxation process. There are many yoga nidra meditation scripts and videos available online that are free to download and listen to. But to give you a taste of this powerful form of relaxation, I have written a simple, short example that I suggest you read and become familiar with and then practise. You might even like to lie on your bed as you do it, and with luck, perhaps you'll just drift off in a way you never have before.

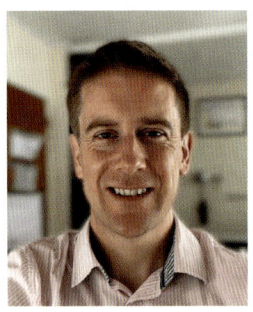

PROFESSIONAL ADVICE

DR MATTHEW ROBINSON
GENERAL PRACTITIONER

Matthew says: 'Looking after our mental health becomes increasingly important as we get older, with depression and dementia being particular problems. While there is little we can do about some of the risk factors for these conditions, we know that regular exercise increases our resilience to stress, improves our sleep and, specifically, that it can reduce the risk of both depression and dementia by up to 30 per cent as well as helping to keep us active and independent.'

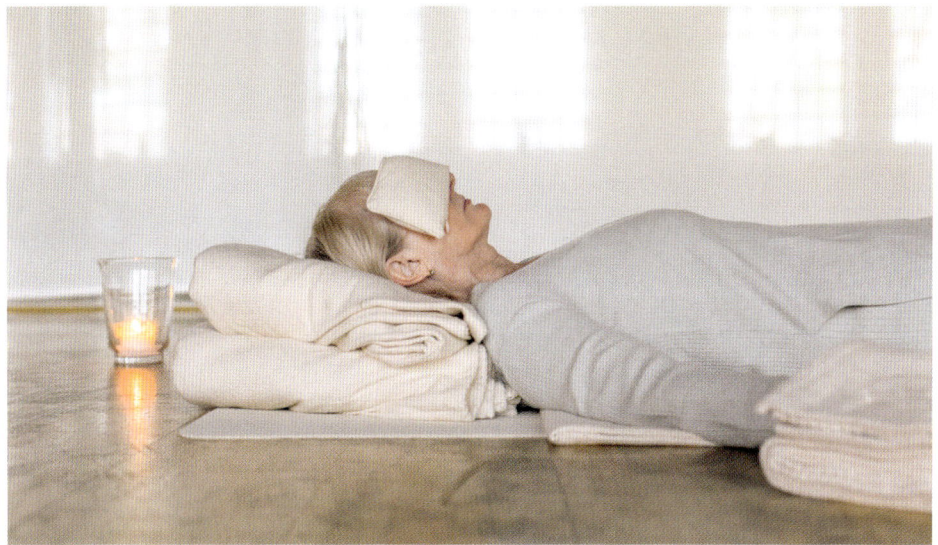

RESTORATIVE YOGA

LEGS ON PILLOW OR CHAIR

Benefits

For this restorative pose, you will use either your chair or a pile of pillows as a prop, depending on your ability. Although this book is Chair Pilates and Yoga and the exercises are in the main performed seated, just for this one posture you will need to lie on your back on the floor with your legs up on your chair or propped up on pillows. If you struggle to get up off the floor once down there, make sure you have something nearby that might help you to get back up to standing. Alternatively, after the relaxation is over, roll on to your front and then on to your hands and knees. From here, use the seat of the chair for support and ease yourself back up to a standing position.

If you suffer from swollen ankles or tired legs, this can be an effective way to alleviate those symptoms. It will also help relieve lower back, hip and knee pain. Before you begin, make sure you can stay warm throughout. Listen to your body and if you find the allotted time is too much, then come out of the pose sooner and do what works for you.

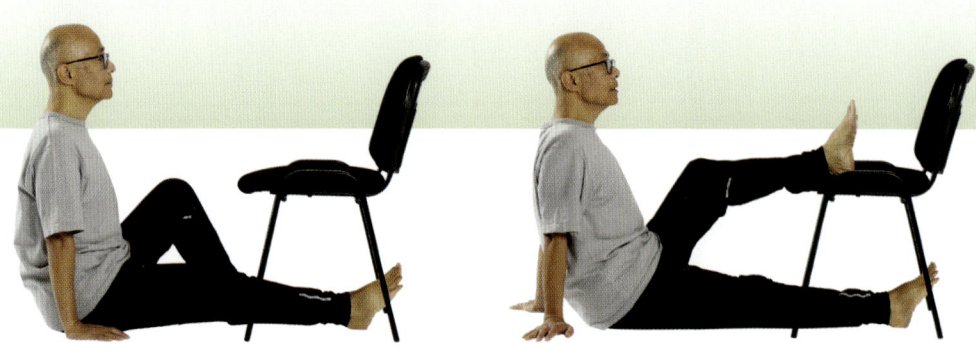

CHAIR VERSION

Method

Single leg

- Start by sitting facing your chair with bent knees.
- Lengthen your right leg out in between the legs of your chair.
- Put your hands, palms down, beside your hips, and gently raise your left leg up on to the chair seat.
- Lie down on your back with your arms relaxed by your sides, palms facing upwards.
- Close your eyes and begin to observe your breathing: in through the nose and out through the nose or mouth. Feel your torso sink into the floor and allow yourself to just let go.
- Stay in this position for 10 minutes, then swap legs.
- After this, remove your knee from the chair, gently roll yourself on to your side and push yourself up to a sitting position.

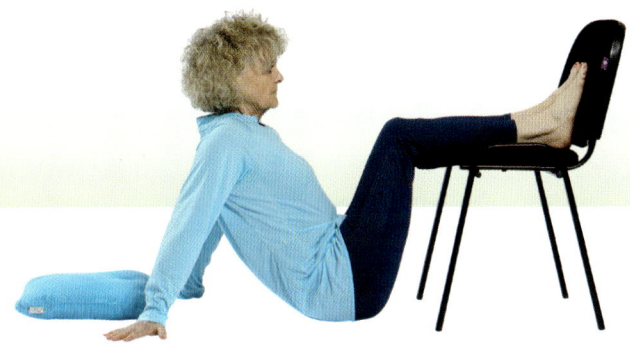

Both legs on the chair

- Start by sitting facing your chair with bent knees.
- Supported by your hands, draw both legs (calves) up on to the seat.
- Lie down on your back with your arms relaxed, palms facing up by your sides.
- Once you are in position, keep your palms facing upwards and legs relaxed and in position, then close your eyes and let your torso sink into the ground.
- Observe your breathing for a moment: feel the air going in through your nostrils and out through your nostrils or mouth, releasing any physical tension that you might be holding on to.
- There is nothing else to do. Just breathe and relax.
- Aim to stay in this position for a minimum of 10 minutes.
- When you feel ready, gently bring your knees towards your chest and roll to one side, pushing yourself up to a sitting position.

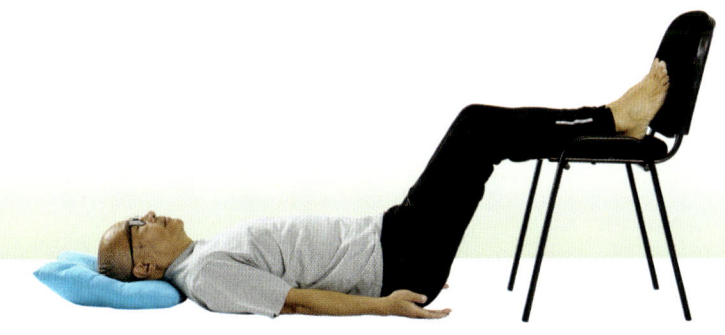

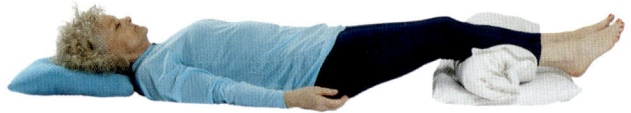

PILLOW VERSION

An alternative to using the chair, and if you find that position hard to manoeuvre yourself into and awkward, then find some pillows from your bed or sofa and pile them up, maybe one or two to start with, and place your lower legs over the top of them.

If it's easier to perform this while lying on your bed with your legs over the pillows, then give that a go. But wherever you choose to practise this, make sure you are comfortable and keep warm. When we relax, our body temperature can drop, so you might like to cover yourself with a blanket.

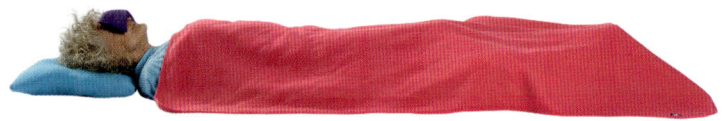

YOGA NIDRA

It's up to you whether you choose to lie on the floor for this short practice or lie on your bed if that is more comfortable for you, or you can stay seated in your chair.

Whatever position you choose, make sure to keep yourself warm; cover yourself with a blanket if you need to. Some people like to cover their eyes as well. You can use an eye pillow if you have one, or a face flannel works well. This will encourage deep relaxation and reduce light exposure. I suggest you familiarise yourself with the following text and then you'll be able to take yourself through it. Alternatively, and if you have the means, record yourself reading the text, pausing between each paragraph and speaking slowly, and then play it back to yourself while lying in the relaxation pose or sitting on your chair.

As already mentioned, you can find many pre-recorded sessions online, so once you understand the process as set out opposite, you might like to find one and play it while you relax.

If you're seated, make sure you feel well supported and comfortable with no distractions. If you are lying down, you might put something under your head to keep your head and spine aligned.

Method

- Close your eyes and scan your body – feet, legs, hips, abdomen, hands, arms, back, shoulders, face, jaw. Just take yourself on a little journey through your body checking for tension or any niggles. Experience any sensations that you might find and allow yourself to settle and begin to relax.
- Breathe in, feel your ribcage expand and then breathe out, letting go of your day and its activities. Let go of any worries that might have been crowding your mind. This is your time; there is nothing else for you to do.
- Let go and rest. Breathing in, breathing out.
- Your thoughts will come and go, which is fine. Feelings might pop up; let them be but without judging or changing them. Allow them to come and go like clouds in the sky floating in and floating away on a gentle breeze.
- Breathe in, noticing your abdomen rising. Breathe out, noticing your abdomen falling.
- Breathe in, noticing your chest rising. Breathe out, noticing your chest falling.

- Your breath is like a wave, rising and falling, rising and falling.
- Now bring your awareness to certain points in your body.
- Starting at the top of your head; your scalp.
- Your forehead.
- Your eyes.
- Your nose; your nostrils.
- Your mouth.
- Your jaw.
- Your neck.
- Your right shoulder; your right elbow; your right wrist; your right hand and fingers, your thumb.
- Breathing in, breathing out.
- Bring your awareness back to your right wrist; right elbow; right shoulder.
- Your chest.
- Your left shoulder; your left elbow; your left wrist; your left wrist and fingers and thumb.
- Breathing in, breathing out.
- Bring your awareness back to your left wrist; your left elbow; your left shoulder.
- Your chest.
- Your upper back.
- Your abdomen: feel the rise and fall of your abdomen as you breathe in and out.
- Your pelvis.
- Your lower back.
- The top of your right leg; your right knee; your right ankle; your foot; your toes; your big toe.

'A body free from nervous tension and fatigue is the ideal shelter provided by nature for housing a well-balanced mind, fully capable of successfully meeting all the complex problems of modern living.'

Joseph Pilates

- Breathing in, breathing out; the calmness of your breath.
- Your right ankle; your right knee; the top of your right leg.
- The top of your left leg; your left knee; your left ankle; your foot; your toes; your big toe.
- Breathing in, breathing out, feeling relaxed.
- Feel your whole body sinking down and letting go.
- Feel calm and at peace.
- Breathing in, breathing out.
- When you are ready, open your eyes and bring yourself back into your room ... if you haven't fallen asleep!
- Notice how you feel.

MINDFUL BREATHING

Benefits

As already mentioned, we tend to take our breathing for granted. But by learning to breathe mindfully, we can calm ourselves both physically and mentally, become more self-aware and reduce stress.

You can do this short breathing exercise either sitting on your chair or lying down on your sofa or bed, but make sure you have no distractions.

Method

- If you're sitting on your chair, sit up tall and lengthen through the spine – you want to remain relaxed but alert.
- Rest your hands on your thighs, relaxing your arms and shoulders.
- If you're happy to do so, close your eyes and take a moment to just be.
- Begin to observe your breath: the gentle inhale through the nose and exhale through your mouth.
- When you feel ready, count a silent one when you breathe in and a silent two when you slowly breathe out through your mouth.

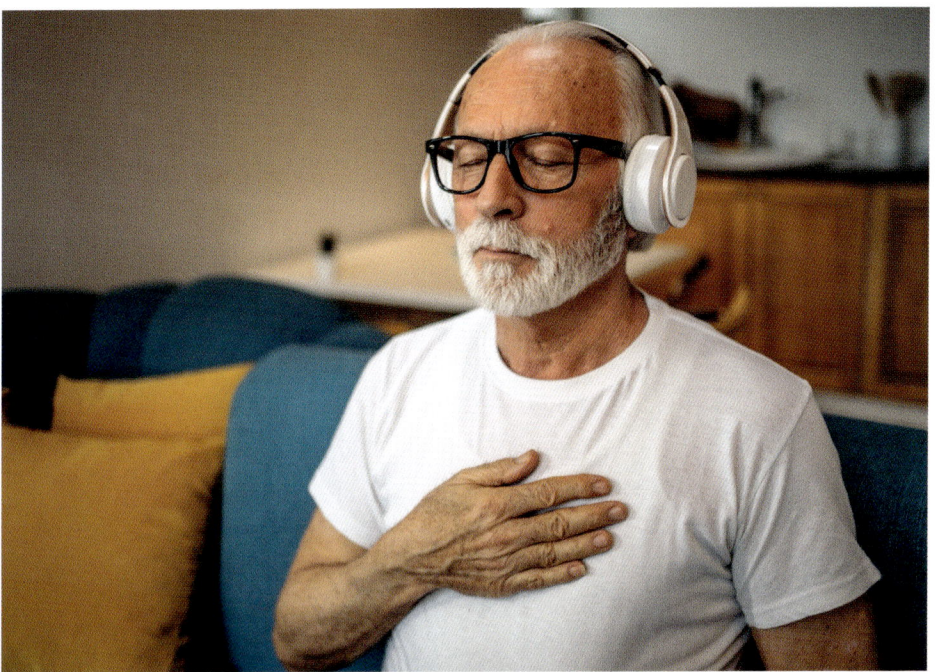

- Count three when you breathe in again, four when you breathe out and so on.
- Continue doing this for as long as you feel you can, maybe a few minutes to start with; you could always set a timer if that helps. Keep the breathing slow and gentle.
- If you find that the chitter-chatter in your head won't quiet and your shopping list or an unresolved problem pops up, that's fine; just let your thoughts come and go and continue to silently count.
- Or you could try this: breathe in slowly for a silent count of three and then breathe out through your mouth for a silent count of six. If you make your exhale longer than your inhale, it can calm your thoughts and even lower your heart rate.

Sleep well!

When the breath wanders the mind is unsteady, but when the breath is calmed, the mind too will be still.'

Svātmārāma, *Hatha Yoga Pradipika*

CHAPTER 22

SEATED DESK WORKOUT

Whatever your age and fitness level, life today often sees us sitting in front of a computer. If you find yourself sitting at a desk all day, then the following suggested exercises are for you — they're very quick and simple and you could make a promise to yourself that you will perform a few of them every couple of hours.

You are already sitting in your chair, so all you need to do is make sure you have enough space around you and get going. Many of the exercises in this book can be performed while at your desk; you just need to turn to the page number of each suggestion. Here are a few suggestions to start you off that include hand and wrist exercises for tired keyboard fingers and some others that aren't seated but can easily be performed at your desk, if you have space. Perfect for that low point in your working day when you begin to feel sluggish.

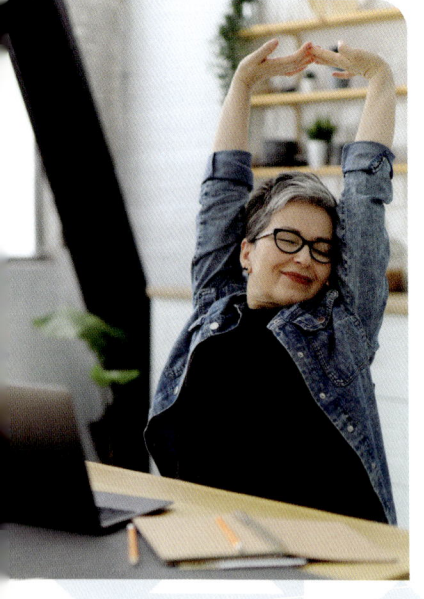

Wake-up Stretches (pp. 44–5) — this is a wonderful and very simple way to release tension if you've been sat at your desk all day working. In fact you might find you already do this automatically every now and again. Perform just a few stretches and some deep breaths every half an hour — you could even set an alarm to remind yourself.

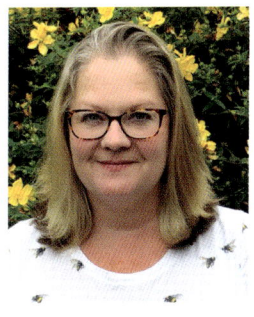

CASE STUDY

VERITY WEST
AGE 45

'I was pretty sceptical at first when I heard about Chair Pilates and Yoga, however I gave some sessions a go and discovered the movements were a really useful alternative exercise technique as I suffer from long-term illness-related fatigue and aches and pains. When I'm feeling like I'm not up to participating in a usual class, attending the Chair Pilates and Yoga sessions helps me to stretch out and strengthen muscles, within a comfortable level for me, whilst still feeling like I'm doing good things for my body. It's also a great way to quickly relieve the stiffness from working at a desk and staring at a screen for long periods of time, which I do too often when working from home.'

Roll Down (pp. 46–7) — you'd need to move your chair away from your desk to perform the roll down but this will lengthen out those stiff back muscles that have been stuck in one position for a while, particularly your lower back.

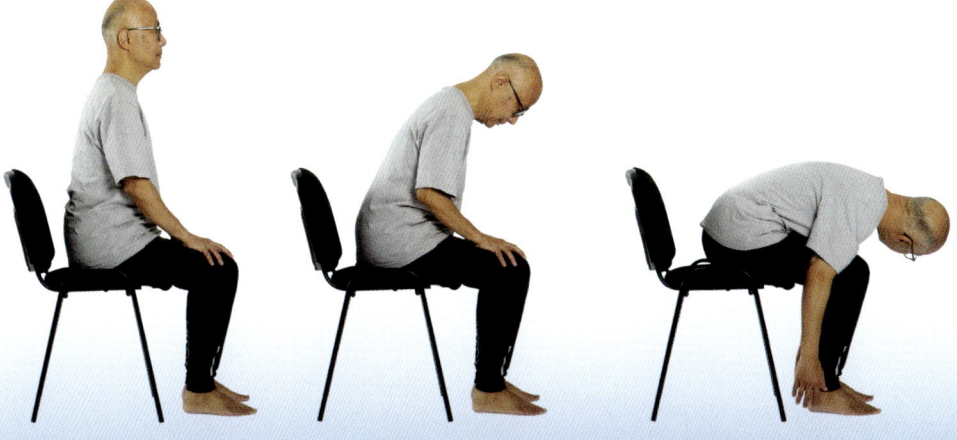

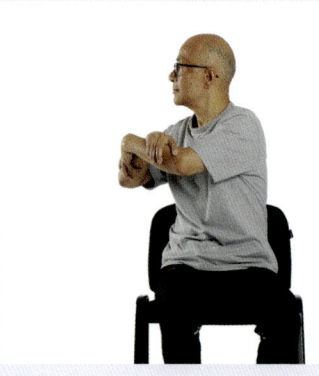

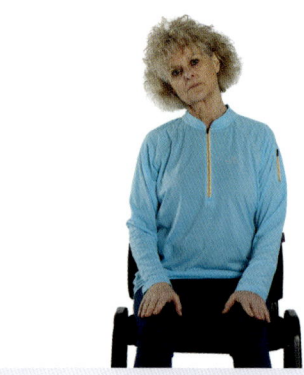

Spinal Rotation (p. 59) — a gentle twist might be all you need to wake yourself up when you've been staring at your computer for hours and sitting in one position without moving your body.

Side neck stretches (p. 51) — the neck can become particularly stiff when sitting at a desk. Depending on your seated posture (slouched, lopsided) and whether you are right or left-handed, you might find one side of your neck is stiffer than the other.

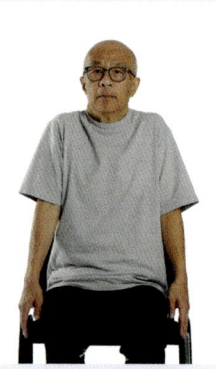

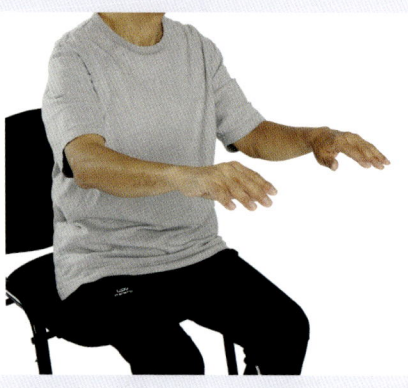

Shoulder Rolls (pp. 54–5) — easy, quick release of any shoulder tension that might have built up.

Piano playing (p. 65) — tired keyboard fingers can benefit from playing the piano and clenching and releasing the hand to relieve tension.

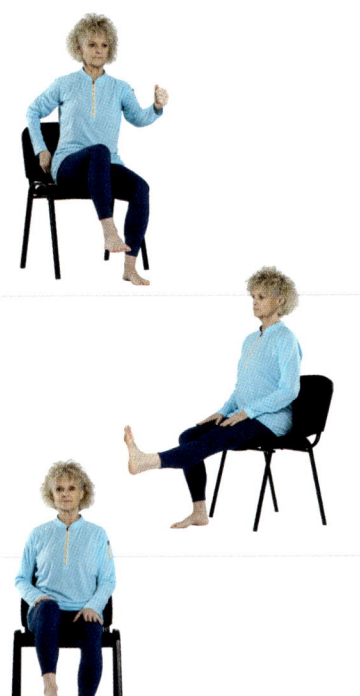

Knee Lifts and Marching Arms and Legs (pp. 99 and 100—1) – sitting still for long lengths of time can produce achy hips and knees, so get them moving – you can even perform these exercises while reading your screen!

Leg Extensions (p. 102) – for tired, sat upon thighs. Sitting weakens the thigh muscles and so performing this exercise from time to time during your working day will keep them functioning well. You'll need to move a little way away from your desk so that you don't kick anything.

Butt Clenches (pp. 94—5) – once again, the more you sit, the weaker your glute muscles will become. This exercise can be easily performed on the hour every hour, throughout your working day.

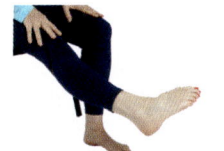

Ankle Mobility (p. 121) – simple and quick, rotate those ankles first one way and then the other way and perhaps include flexing and pointing of the toes as well.

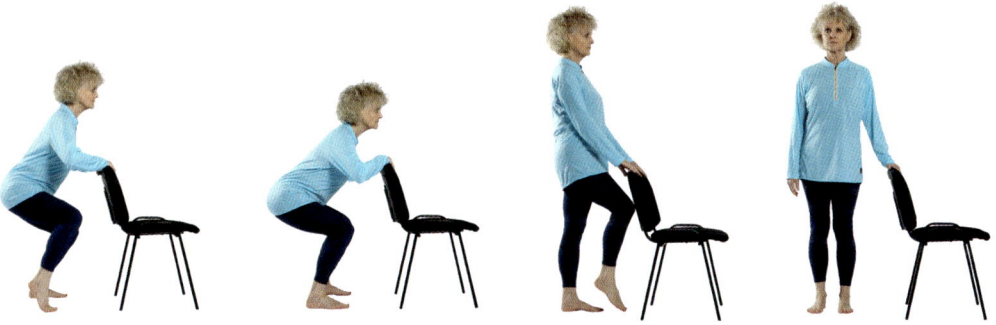

Calf Raises Balance, Squat and Balance 1 and 2 (pp. 139, 138, 133, 134) – using your chair as a prop (but if it has wheels, please make sure that it is locked).

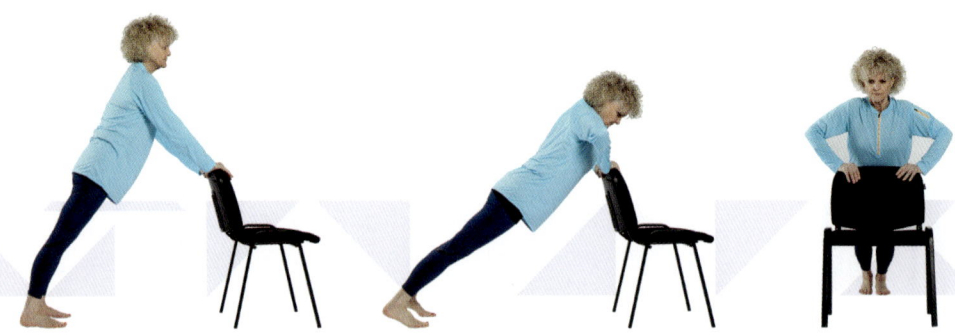

EXTRA

CHAIR OR DESK PUSH-UP

Method

- Face your chair or desk and place the palms of your hands flat on top with your arms slightly wider than your shoulders and your arms straight.
- Take a step back.
- Take a breath in and as you breathe out, lower your torso until your chest nearly reaches your chair or desk.
- Breathe in again and as you breathe out, push yourself back up. Try to keep your spine straight and your neck in line with your spine.
- Repeat 8 times or as many times as you feel able, progressing to more repetitions.

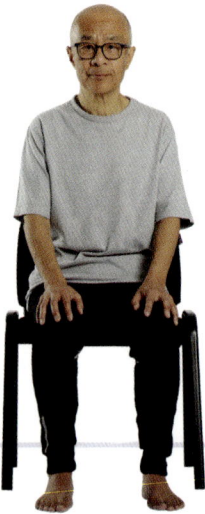

Mindful Breathing (p. 178) – perfect for stressful office meetings! Although perhaps not during them but before or after!

CHAPTER 23

SHORT ROUTINES

BEGINNER

A simple session that moves the whole body to start you off. These are just suggestions and once you're familiar with other exercises, you can mix and match your own routines, finding what works best for you.

Warm up

Breathing and Body Scan (p. 43)

Wake-up Stretches (p. 44)

Roll Down (p. 46)

Side Neck Stretches (p. 51)

Shoulder Rolls (pp. 54—5)

Upper body

Piano Playing Fingers (p. 65)

Biceps (pp. 70—1)

Triceps (p. 73)

Deltoids (pp. 74—5)

Cactus Arms (p. 76)

Scissor Arms (p. 77)

Lower body

Heel Slides (p. 97)

Knee Lifts (p. 99)

Treacle feet (p. 100)

Marching Arms and Legs (p. 101)

Cushion Squeeze (p. 109)

Foot Pedalling (pp. 114—5)

Ankle Mobility (p. 121)

Toe Curls and Toe Yoga (pp. 119—20)

Sit to stand and balance

Sit to Stand, Version 1 (p. 128)

Balance 1 (p. 133)

To finish

Upper Back Stretch (p. 164)

Facial Exercises (from p. 125)

Mindful Breathing (p. 178)

INTERMEDIATE

A simple intermediate session to get you started. These are just suggestions and once you're familiar with other exercises, you can mix and match your own routines.

Warm-up

Breathing and Body Scan (p. 43)

Wake-up Stretches (p. 44)

Roll Down (p. 46)

Side Neck Stretches (p. 51)

Shoulder Rolls (pp. 54–5)

Upper body

Shoulder and Arm Rotations (pp. 54–5)

Number 8, Garden Gate (p. 79)

Row, Row, Row (p. 83)

Pack a Punch 2 (p. 85)

Piano Playing Fingers (p. 65)

Abdominals

Sit-up and Crunch Time (pp. 90–1)

Crunch Time 2 (p. 91)

Lower Abdominal Muscles (p. 92)

Obliques (p. 89)

Lower body

Knee Lifts (p. 99)

Marching Arms and Legs (p. 100–01)

Leg Extensions (p. 102)

Mix and Match Leg Kicks (p. 103)

Knee to Elbow Rotation (p. 104)

Hip Opener (pp. 106–7)

Hippy, Hippy Shake (p. 108)

Cross Legs (p. 111)

Toe Yoga (p. 120)

Sit to stand and balance

Sit to Stand, Version 2 (p. 129)

Balance 3 (p. 135)

To finish

Triangle (p. 166)

Facial Exercises (from p. 125)

Mindful Breathing (p. 178)

Though no one can go back and make a brand new start, anyone can start from now and make a brand new ending.'

Carl Bard

REFERENCES

Introduction

'NHS guidelines state that for those of us over 65…': 'Physical activity guidelines for older adults', NHS: https://www.nhs.uk/live-well/exercise/exercise-guidelines/physical-activity-guidelines-older-adults/.

Chapter 1

'we lose approximately 3–8 per cent of our muscle mass …': Volpi, E., Nazemi, R. and Fujita, S., 'Muscle tissue changes with aging', National Library of Medicine: https://www.ncbi.nlm.nih.gov/pmc/articles/PMC2804956.

'The proportion of people who are physically inactive increases sharply with age': 'The State of Ageing 2022', Centre for Ageing Better: https://ageing-better.org.uk/health-state-ageing-2022.

Chapter 4

'According to a report by the National Heart, Lung and Blood Institute, good hydration is linked to healthy ageing…': 'Good hydration linked to healthy aging', National Heart, Lung and Blood Institute: https://www.nhlbi.nih.gov/news/2023/good-hydration-linked-healthy-aging.

'According to the National Center for Health Research, music can make for a more enjoyable workout.': Markell, J., 'Can Listening to Music Improve Your Workout?', National Centre for Health Research: https://www.center4research.org/can-listening-music-improve-workout.

Chapter 6

'More than 85% of people over the age of 60 are affected [by Cervical spondylosis]': 'Cervical Spondylosis (Arthritis of the Neck)', OrthoInfo: https://orthoinfo.aaos.org/en/diseases--conditions/cervical-spondylosis-arthritis-of-the-neck.

Chapter 9

'A research study published in *The Lancet* in 2015 demonstrated that rheumatoid arthritis sufferers ...': '9 Exercises to Help Hand Arthritis', Arthritis Foundation: https://www.arthritis.org/health-wellness/healthy-living/physical-activity/other-activities/9-exercises-to-help-hand-arthritis.

Chapter 10

'A journal article in *Age and Ageing* published by Oxford University Press ...': Marion, E., McMurdo, T., Rennie, L., 'A Controlled Trial of Exercise by Residents of Old People's Homes', *Age and Ageing*: https://academic.oup.com/ageing/article-abstract/22/1/11/14852.

Chapter 15

'...facial exercises can indeed go some way to helping our facial appearance.': Alam, M., Walter, A. J., Geisler, A., et al, 'Association of Facial Exercise With the Appearance of Aging', Jama Dermatology, available at National Library of Medicine: https://www.ncbi.nlm.nih.gov/pmc/articles/PMC5885810/.

Chapter 21

'It is estimated that between 40 and 70 per cent of older adults sleep badly.': Miner, B. and Kryger, M. H., 'Sleep in the Aging Population', National Library of Medicine: https://pubmed.ncbi.nlm.nih.gov/28159095/.

INDEX

Exercises marked (B) are Beginner and (I) are Intermediate

ACKNOWLEDGEMENTS

Thank you to all my clients who contributed to this book, particularly Molly who persuaded me to start a regular seated exercise session. And thank you to Dame Sheila Hancock for writing such kind words about Chair Pilates and Yoga. Thanks go to my local Age UK group in Marlow and its guests, who were a joy to teach and talk with about their exercise routines, or lack of them! Thank you to the experts Dr Helen Kennedy, Dr Matthew Robinson, Jane Kaushal and Sara Carter, and finally, thank you to Charlotte, Megan and the team at Bloomsbury for their support.

ABOUT THE AUTHOR

Harri has worked in the fitness industry for over 30 years and teaches Pilates and yoga. She's passionate about ageing successfully, helping the unfit get fit, and encouraging people to find time to step outside and enjoy the healing power of nature. When she's not teaching, running or walking on trails, she likes to crochet or write. Harri has written two other books, _Pilates for Runners_ and _Pilates for Living_, both published by Bloomsbury.